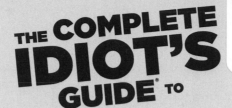

D0599290

Hormone Weight Loss

by Alicia Stanton, M.D.

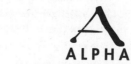

A member of Penguin Group (USA) Inc.

This book is dedicated to Al and Ginny Stanton, my parents, who have always been the wind beneath my wings. I love you!

ALPHA BOOKS

Published by the Penguin Group

Penguin Group (USA) Inc., 375 Hudson Street, New York, New York 10014, USA

Penguin Group (Canada), 90 Eglinton Avenue East, Suite 700, Toronto, Ontario M4P 2Y3, Canada (a division of Pearson Penguin Canada Inc.)

Penguin Books Ltd., 80 Strand, London WC2R 0RL, England

Penguin Ireland, 25 St. Stephen's Green, Dublin 2, Ireland (a division of Penguin Books Ltd.)

Penguin Group (Australia), 250 Camberwell Road, Camberwell, Victoria 3124, Australia (a division of Pearson Australia Group Pty. Ltd.)

Penguin Books India Pvt. Ltd., 11 Community Centre, Panchsheel Park, New Delhi—110 017, India

Penguin Group (NZ), 67 Apollo Drive, Rosedale, North Shore, Auckland 1311, New Zealand (a division of Pearson New Zealand Ltd.)

Penguin Books (South Africa) (Pty.) Ltd., 24 Sturdee Avenue, Rosebank, Johannesburg 2196, South Africa

Penguin Books Ltd., Registered Offices: 80 Strand, London WC2R 0RL, England

International Standard Book Number: 978-1-61564-102-4
Library of Congress Catalog Card Number: 2010917072

13 12   8 7 6 5 4 3 2

Interpretation of the printing code: The rightmost number of the first series of numbers is the year of the book's printing; the rightmost number of the second series of numbers is the number of the book's printing. For example, a printing code of 11-1 shows that the first printing occurred in 2011.

Printed in the United States of America

Note: This publication contains the opinions and ideas of its author. It is intended to provide helpful and informative material on the subject matter covered. It is sold with the understanding that the author and publisher are not engaged in rendering professional services in the book. If the reader requires personal assistance or advice, a competent professional should be consulted.

The author and publisher specifically disclaim any responsibility for any liability, loss, or risk, personal or otherwise, which is incurred as a consequence, directly or indirectly, of the use and application of any of the contents of this book.

Most Alpha books are available at special quantity discounts for bulk purchases for sales promotions, premiums, fund-raising, or educational use. Special books, or book excerpts, can also be created to fit specific needs.

For details, write: Special Markets, Alpha Books, 375 Hudson Street, New York, NY 10014.

Publisher: *Marie Butler-Knight*

Associate Publisher: *Mike Sanders*

Executive Managing Editor: *Billy Fields*

Acquisitions Editor: *Tom Stevens*

Development Editor: *Ginny Bess Munroe*

Senior Production Editor: *Kayla Dugger*

Copy Editor: *Kelly Henthorne*

Cover Designer: *Kurt Owens*

Book Designers: *William Thomas, Rebecca Batchelor*

Indexer: *Heather McNeill*

Layout: *Ayanna Lacey*

Proofreader: *John Etchison*

Contents

Introduction

We live in truly amazing times. Every day we see new technological advances in every aspect of our lives: medicine, communication, travel, entertainment, and many others. However, in a time when we are moving forward in so many areas, why are we struggling so much with our health? Obesity has reached epidemic proportions. Heart disease, diabetes, cancer, autoimmune disease, Alzheimer's, and many other chronic diseases continue to plague us. Many of these diseases have some relationship to obesity.

As a physician, it's very difficult for me to watch patients struggling with weight gain, fatigue, low sex drive, difficulty sleeping, and mood changes who've been told by other physicians that "you are just getting older" or "your laboratory values are in the normal range so there is nothing wrong with you." The reality is that many of our technological advances have put us in a situation where our metabolism is being damaged. Damage to your metabolism sets you up to easily gain weight, then have great difficulty taking it back off. The driving force behind your metabolism is your hormones.

I have been focusing on the nutritional and hormonal balance of my patients for over 10 years. Originally, I underwent the "standard" medical school training, which meant that I had very little appreciation for the role of nutrition in disease. Of course, I knew about rare things like scurvy, rickets, and beriberi—diseases of extreme vitamin deficiency. However, I didn't truly understand the all-encompassing effect that diet had on metabolism and on overall health. Hippocrates, the father of medicine, said it best when he said, "Let your food be your medicine."

My journey started back in 1997. I was very happy practicing in my OB/GYN practice and being the mother to my 18-month-old son, Eric. My life was turned upside down one day in October when, after experiencing back pain and visiting my physician, I was diagnosed with a spinal cord tumor. The tumor was not aggressive and was surgically removed four days later. However, surgery left me temporarily paralyzed from the waist down and in chronic pain. With therapy, I regained the use of my legs and was able to return to my practice in a few months. But my life was very different. I began to research ways, besides pain medication, to help me cope with the pain. At that point, I discovered acupuncture, massage, and osteopathy as excellent ways to alleviate pain. More importantly, I learned that these things worked better if my nutrition was good.

I began to study the effects of nutrition in medicine with the American Academy of Anti-Aging. I learned more about nutrition and began to understand its importance in relation to metabolism, hormone balance, and disease. This began my quest to understand as much as I could about these relationships. As I began implementing my knowledge, I began to feel much better. Then I started using the things I learned to help me to start helping my patients. I talked to them about their diets, their sleep habits, and their levels of stress. I began diagnosing hormone imbalance and treating with diet, lifestyle changes, and, when necessary, bioidentical hormone therapy.

I noticed drastic improvements in the health of my patients as we began focusing on true prevention of disease rather than just treating their symptoms. They lost weight, they slept better, they had better sex, and they were happier in general. Eventually, I closed the OB/GYN practice and opened a practice that focuses solely on hormone balance and nutrition.

One of the biggest problems with our current medical system is that we tend to focus on medications to treat symptoms of diseases rather than looking at the causes of those diseases. Many times, the thought process is, once you're on medication for something like high blood pressure or high cholesterol, you're on it for life. These medications are not without their own side effects. Often, you might get a side effect from one medication and be put on another medication to help with a side effect of the first one. The risk of drug interactions increases with every medication that is added to the list.

When you really start understanding the delicate balance of our hormones and their influence on our metabolism, it's easy to see how using medications only to treat symptoms can become a recipe for disaster. I definitely believe the medications have a place in patient treatment. However, I also believe that we have great power to manage our health and keep our hormones balanced by the way we eat, sleep, manage stress, and eliminate toxins every day.

First of all, you have to understand how all of these relationships work. Why does it matter if you eat white bread and candy instead of apples and green beans? If you can get by on five hours of sleep a night, why shouldn't you? You're eating almost no fat and no cholesterol, yet you continue to gain weight and your cholesterol keeps going up; what's up with that? You try diet after diet and exercise plan after exercise plan, yet the scale never seems to move or, worse yet, it moves up; why? If you have any of these questions, this book has the answers.

This book is the culmination of years of experience with thousands of patients. As I've worked with these patients, I have found that seven basic principles can be used to create hormone balance, a healthy metabolism, and weight loss. Not only do I help you understand these principles, I give you the tools to put them into practice in your daily life. As you utilize these principles and balance your metabolism, you'll find that you lose weight, flatten your belly, sleep better, have more energy, build more muscle, have better sex, and feel better in general.

In this book, I teach you what to eat and what to eliminate from your diet. Not only will you have step-by-step instructions, I have included meal suggestions, 56 days' worth of menus, and a number of excellent recipes. In addition, you'll learn what toxins you encounter in everyday life and how to avoid them. I show you how to use the fastest and most efficient ways to burn fat and build muscle. The truth is, you don't have to spend hours in the gym every day. Everyone knows that it's important to reduce stress; I will show you the hidden sources of stress you may not know about and exactly what to do to relieve stress. You'll also learn which supplements might be important for you and how to shop for them.

At the end of the day, we have much more control over our health and well-being than we think we do. The first step is understanding what has happened and why so many of us are having so much trouble with hormone balance and weight gain. The next step is implementing all of the things you learned into your life so you can fine-tune your hormones, heal your metabolism, lose the weight you want to, and live a much healthier life.

What's in This Book

This book is made up of four parts:

Part 1, From Unhealthy to Healthy Hormones, helps you understand the many factors that are contributing to our current obesity epidemic. I also review 10 of the hormones that are related to weight and what each of the hormones does. When you understand these hormone connections, you can use that knowledge to apply the seven principles for hormone weight loss to your everyday life.

Part 2, Losing Weight with Healthy Hormones, provides details for all seven principles of the hormone weight-loss diet. Each of the principles focuses on a specific aspect of how you can change your diet and lifestyle to balance your hormones and lose weight. I include a lot of great information, quotes, and tips to help you see how all these things are connected.

Part 3, Putting the Principles into Action, is literally the how-to section. You learn specifically how the hormone weight-loss diet works, what you should eat, and what you should avoid. You also learn the specifics of how you can avoid toxins in your everyday life. Your body needs a lot of different vitamins and nutrients to create energy, burn calories, and help you lose weight. I review some of the more important supplements to aid in weight loss. I also have a quiz you can take to see what possible hormone imbalances you may have.

Besides diet, exercise is thought of as a key component of weight loss. I'll show you the best kinds of exercises to do to help increase your lean muscle mass, burn fat, and balance your hormones. Two of the unsung heroes in weight loss are stress reduction and sleep. I give you a number of tips and supplement suggestions to really improve your sleep. In addition, I provide you with the explanations for a number of possible stress reduction techniques, some of which you can do anywhere!

Part 4, Continuing Success, gives you the framework to design your personal action plan for hormone balance and weight loss, with information specifically tailored to children, teens, men, women, and seniors. The action plan is supplemented with worksheets that allow you to track your daily progress. This is important because studies show that tracking your food intake and exercise contributes to an increase in weight loss and more success in keeping the weight off. In addition, you'll track your exercise results and measurements, which will allow you to clearly see your progress.

I provide a large number of meal suggestions and food tables listing the different foods that are allowed in a format that lets you mix and match the foods to your own tastes. There are also 28-day menu plans for Phase I and Phase II of the diet with a number of amazing recipes.

In the appendixes, you'll find a glossary of terms, resources on where to locate many of the products, information on supplementation for common health problems, personal action plan worksheets, and the most frequent questions I get, along with my answers.

Extras

Throughout the book, you'll see sidebars that provide additional information. They are:

DID YOU KNOW?

Important facts and statistics related to hormones and weight.

DEFINITION

Definitions related to hormones and weight loss.

THAT'S QUOTABLE

Quotes from experts in the field.

TRUSTY TIP

Helpful tips for you to put the suggestions in the book to use.

Acknowledgments

I am humbled by the number of amazing people that contributed to this book. I love to learn and have such gratitude for those who have been able to teach me, whether it's a scientific lesson or one that gives me deeper understanding of those around me.

To my husband, Robert, who makes every day seem like Christmas morning. Thank you for your patience and belief in me. In the midst of the most difficult times, your smile, your touch, and your love give me all the answers I need.

To my beautiful sons, Eric (age 15) and Evan (age 11), who show me the world from a new vantage point every day. Thank you for supporting me as I wrote this book even though it meant I couldn't spend as much time with you. I've loved you since before you were born and one of the most amazing things in my life is watching you grow to young men.

To my parents, Al and Ginny Stanton, my sister, Amy, my brother, Rob, and the rest of my family, who are the most loving, supportive people I know. Because of you, I have had the ability to develop my talents, spread my wings, and fly.

To my many brilliant mentors, the beauty of sharing your knowledge is that you can give it away to others but you still keep it yourself. Thank you for giving so much of your knowledge and insights to me over the years. I can't name them all, but I want to give special thanks to Dr. Pamela Smith, Dr. Patrick Hanaway, Dr. Mark Hyman, Dr. Stephen Sinatra, Dr. Shari Lieberman, Dr. Jeffrey Bland, Dr. Dan Lukaczer, Dr. Ron Rothenberg, Dr. Jim Lavelle, Dr. Christiane Northrup, Dr. Diana Schwarzbein, and Dr. Andrew Weil.

To Marilyn Allen, my literary agent and my friend, thank you for your excellent work in bringing this project to me. More importantly, thank you for your wisdom, humor, and infinite patience!

To Betsy Vierck, thank you for your insights and your guidance. I really appreciate all that you did to bring this wonderful book together.

To Tom Stevens at Alpha Books, thank you for your patience, wisdom, and guidance. I truly appreciate your belief in me and your willingness to overcome the many obstacles we faced.

To Michelle, Laura, and Shannon at Common Language, thank you for continually jumping in to help out with anything I need. I couldn't ask for a more intelligent, compassionate, and capable group of women to work with.

To Andrew Romeo at CrossFit Revelation, thank you for your guidance with the exercise section of the book. You have given me a whole new way to look at physical fitness, and I am so very grateful!

To Deborah and Kurt, thank you for being my "voice of reason" so many times. You make everything so clear and you mean more to me than I can ever express.

To the Stanton family, the Burns family, Andrew and the Mau family, the BodyLogicMD family, Steven, Kevin, Michelle, Maika, Janis, Tamara, Jeff, Corinne, Glenn, and Debbie, who stuck with me through thick and thin. Thank you for all that you do every day. It truly does "take a village" to help with anyone's success.

To Bill and Steve Harrison, who gave me the knowledge, the spark, and the connections to make my dreams a reality.

Last but most certainly not least, thank you to my patients. It is an honor and privilege to be involved in your lives and your care. I pray that I have given you as much value over the years as you have given to me.

Special Thanks to the Technical Reviewer

The Complete Idiot's Guide to Hormone Weight Loss was reviewed by an expert who double-checked the accuracy of what you'll learn here, to help us ensure that this book gives you everything you need to know about hormones and losing weight. Special thanks are extended to Jeffrey L Thackrey, M.D., M.P.H., Medical Director, BodyLogicMD of Fort Lauderdale.

Trademarks

All terms mentioned in this book that are known to be or are suspected of being trademarks or service marks have been appropriately capitalized. Alpha Books and Penguin Group (USA) Inc. cannot attest to the accuracy of this information. Use of a term in this book should not be regarded as affecting the validity of any trademark or service mark.

From Unhealthy to Healthy Hormones

There are more than 100 hormones in the human body. I describe 10 of the hormones that are related to weight and what each one does. I also list symptoms of hormone imbalance and the causes and conditions related to imbalance.

The chapters in Part 1 help you understand the many factors that are contributing to our current obesity epidemic. Our current diet, loaded with refined carbohydrates, increased sugar consumption, high fructose corn syrup, trans fats, hormones, pesticides, and antibiotics is a part of the problem. However, many of us don't appreciate how hormones can make it much easier to gain weight and much harder to lose it when you've gained it. The problem is compounded further by our high stress levels.

It's important to appreciate the connection between your diet, stress levels, toxin exposures, and hormone balance. What's so important about insulin? Does it matter what our cortisol levels are? How can drinking from plastic water bottles cause me to gain weight? I review 10 of the hormones that are related to weight and what each of the hormones does.

What's the Problem?

In This Chapter

- Why our current diets don't work
- Why the kinds of calories matter more than the number of calories
- How toxins affect our weight
- How insulin resistance works
- Why refined carbohydrates are more problematic than dietary fat

Joan is frustrated. She watches what she eats, tries to exercise, and tries to get enough sleep (often without success). Joan thinks her lifestyle is pretty healthy, but she gained back the 20 pounds she lost last year, and no matter what she does, it won't come off again. "It was much easier to lose weight the first few times," Joan says.

Other problems nag Joan. Every morning she has to hit the snooze button on her alarm two or three times before she can finally get out of bed. Her hair and skin are dry, no matter how much body lotion or hair conditioner she uses. She can't even think about sex; she's too tired.

Joan's doctor has done laboratory tests, which are "normal." She is told that she is getting older and that it wouldn't hurt for her to lose 10 or 15 pounds. The truth is that Joan's hormones are not balanced.

Like Joan, many people suffer from major hormone imbalance, which results in weight gain and many other unpleasant symptoms. This condition is silent. It goes undetected due to a lack of awareness on everyone's part—the sufferer, family, friends, and doctors.

In this chapter, you're introduced to why hormone balance is so important in maintaining a healthy weight and how your hormones are supposed to be balanced. You then look ahead to what you can do to keep your hormones balanced and your weight under control.

Obesity Is Rising

Americans suffer from obesity-related diseases like diabetes (25 million), prediabetes (60 million), metabolic syndrome, hypothyroidism (underactive thyroid), depression, and many other problems. In addition to those diagnosed with these diseases, many more don't feel well but aren't sick enough to warrant a diagnosis. They may not think they are sick enough to go to a doctor, or they do go to a doctor, and the standard laboratory tests like cholesterol, thyroid panels, and blood chemistries most physicians use show "normal" results.

Obesity is rising, and dieting isn't taking care of the problem. Of all the diets that people embark on, only 2 to 6 percent are successful. If the dieter uses calorie restriction to lose weight, the average person ultimately regains any weight lost plus an additional 5 pounds for every diet they go on!

You're told that, in order to lose weight, you must eat less and exercise more. In terms of "calorie math," it does make sense that taking in fewer calories while also exercising to "work off" extra calories results in a calorie deficit, and you will lose weight. However, for many, this approach doesn't work. You know people who eat "almost nothing" and can't lose a single pound. Many times, they're accused of eating more than they are telling others.

In reality, it's not just the number of calories you take in; it's the *type* of calories. As you'll see in the next section, your body handles the calories from sugar and high fructose corn syrup differently than it handles calories from proteins, vegetables, and unsaturated fats.

What Your Genetic Makeup Needs

Our genetic makeup is almost identical to that of our ancestors of 120 million years ago when we lived a hunter-gatherer lifestyle. We survived by hunting game and gathering vegetation for our food. We didn't grow or process it. We did very well for millions of years on whole foods such as fruits, vegetables, lean meats, nuts, and seeds.

Around 10,000 years ago, things changed and we discovered how to grow crops and began an agrarian way of life. One major change was that we began eating the grains we grew. Although this did wonders for our taste buds and food supply, it may have been the beginning of some health problems. Our genes and DNA weren't designed to digest the grains we started growing and eating. As we continue to eat these grains, refine the nutrients out of them, and add processed foods such as trans-fatty acids and high fructose corn syrup, we have seen those health problems amplified in the past 50 years.

In his book *The Paleo Solution*, Robb Wolf recounts the true story about two prehistoric populations that lived near the Ohio River Valley: the farmers (Hardin Village group), who lived 500 years ago, and the hunter-gatherers (Indian Knoll group), who lived 3,000 to 5,000 years ago. The sites are important because each one produced a large number of skeletal remains that could be studied. The diet of the agricultural Hardin Village group was mainly corn, beans, and squash. The diet of the hunter-gatherer Indian Knoll group was meats, fruits, fish, and shellfish. The differences between the two sets of skeletons are striking.

- The hunter-gatherers had almost no cavities, and the farmers had almost 7 cavities per person.

- The hunter-gatherers showed less bone malformations consistent with poor nutrition.

- The hunter-gatherers showed a much lower rate of infant mortality, especially between the ages of 2 and 4, when malnutrition is most damaging to children.

- The hunter-gatherers on average lived longer than the farmers.

- The hunter-gatherers did not show signs of iron, calcium, and protein deficiencies, which were common in the farmers.

One of the key aspects of the hunter-gatherer diet was that it was limited in sugars. It contained animal, fish, and shellfish proteins; fats and proteins from nuts and seeds; and carbohydrates from vegetables and a few fruits (in season). This is a lot different than our current diet, which focuses on grains, many of them processed; sugars; and "fake foods" like high fructose corn syrup, artificial sweeteners, trans fats, and a year-round supply of fruits. As we will see, the sugars and fake foods are a big part of our current obesity crisis.

This is all very interesting, but what does it have to do with our hormones? Because hormones are the messengers throughout our bodies and they must be well balanced in order to function properly, they are susceptible to changes inside our body and in the outside environment.

The major changes in our diet that occurred when society moved from being hunter-gatherers to farmers set us up to consume more sugars and starches, which paved the way for hormone imbalance and an increase in disease. The difference in the health of the two tribes helps us see the trend that was started when we began focusing on a grain-based diet. As we continue to add preservatives, pesticides, and fake foods as we have over the past 50 years, the problems grow exponentially.

You Are What You Eat

The building blocks your body uses to construct its cells, bones, proteins, and other parts come from the food you give it. Biologically speaking, there is a big difference in the structure of the cells of an individual who eats mainly junk food, trans fats, artificial sweeteners, and refined carbohydrates compared to the individual who eats whole foods such as lean meats, vegetables, fruits, nuts, seeds, and healthy fats.

The differences in cell structures create differences in cell functions. In other words, the bottom line is that your body is not going to work as well if its cells are constructed from junk materials as it would if the diet that supported it consisted of high-quality nutritional sources.

Processed Foods

Processed foods are among the worst offenders. The major components of processed foods are corn, wheat, and soy, which have been turned into wheat flour, partially hydrogenated corn oil, and hydrolyzed soy protein. Because they don't retain many of their natural qualities, our bodies no longer recognize them as foods, which leads to hormone imbalance and weight gain. In fact, most processed foods should be called *body fill* (as in "land fill") and they should not be referred to as foods at all.

> **DEFINITION**
>
> **Body fill** is any food that does not provide adequate nutritional value to help cells grow or reactions in the body run efficiently. The worst offenders actually create problems for the body such as inflammation or damage to the arteries.

Adding insult to injury, because wheat, soy, and corn by themselves don't have that much flavor, the food manufacturer adds fat and sugar to improve the taste. These additives trick our brains into wanting more. How does this work? Foods that are high in fat and sugar cause the release of opioids from the brain, which is our bodies' natural form of the feel-good drug morphine. We feel great when we eat these foods, and it's easy to get addicted.

High Fructose Corn Syrup

The man-made chemical called high fructose corn syrup is another derivative of corn. It's found in almost every processed or packaged food and most of the fast foods people consume every day. It has no vitamins, minerals, antioxidants, proteins, essential fats, or fiber. What it does have is "empty calories," which taste great, but make people fat!

High fructose corn syrup wasn't in our food supply as recently as the 1970s. Now it's used to sweeten thousands of foods and drinks. Our current consumption of sodas averages 54 gallons per person per year. That is a lot of high fructose corn syrup!

DID YOU KNOW?

A can of soda has about 40 grams of high fructose corn syrup, equivalent to about 9 teaspoons of sugar. That's why many nutritionists call soda "liquid candy."

The sad story of high fructose corn syrup doesn't end with the fact that it's ubiquitous and full of empty calories. Consumption of the syrup stresses the liver and actually makes us hungrier for more sweets. As I talked about earlier, the increased levels of sugar in our bodies are creating many of our obesity problems.

One of the major problems with high sugar in our bloodstream is that the hormone insulin is needed to help you move the sugar from your bloodstream and into your cells. Insulin is a lifesaving hormone because it helps you get the energy your cells need from the bloodstream. However, when you constantly eat foods high in sugar, you have a lot of sugar in your bloodstream all the time, which means you must constantly call on insulin to move the sugar from your bloodstream to the cells.

Other Food Additives

In addition to the fats and sugars that are added to processed foods, manufacturers also add artificial colors and preservatives. One such preservative, butylated hydroxy-anisole (BHA), is categorized as "generally recognized as safe" by the FDA. However, it is a known "endocrine disruptor," which means it creates hormone imbalance either by mimicking a hormone or blocking it. If a hormone is mimicked, the body may think that there is too much of it present. On the other hand, if it's blocked, the body might be missing it.

In this case, BHA appears to block testosterone and thyroid. Testosterone is very important for building muscle and, as you will learn in later chapters, the more muscle you have, the higher your metabolism. Thyroid hormone is also important for maintaining a healthy metabolism. Therefore, blocking these hormones can easily lead to weight gain.

TRUSTY TIP

To limit your exposure to BHA, limit your intake of processed foods. Whole foods don't need preservatives such as BHA.

BHA is found in hundreds of our foods, beverages, cosmetics, and skin care products. Keep in mind that many of the things we rub onto our skin are absorbed into our bodies. By eating these preservatives in our foods and rubbing them onto our skin, we ingest large doses of it every day. The more we take in, the higher our risk of endocrine disruption. It's interesting to note that some safer substances, such as vitamin E, could replace BHA to preserve our foods.

Insulin and the Pizza Man

Your weight is influenced by a number of hormones, one of which is insulin. It puts nutrients into your cells. However, if insulin is not well balanced and is present in high levels in your body, it can contribute significantly to weight gain.

Why? In order for your body to use food as fuel for energy, the digested food is broken down and enters your bloodstream as sugar, or glucose. When this process is well balanced, you have a constant level of energy available to your cells and adequate energy storage to use if needed. Insulin is an important part of this process. It moves glucose to cells where, in the case of muscle cells, it can generate energy. The bad news is that insulin can also move glucose for storage in fat cells.

Different foods are converted into blood glucose at different rates. Refined flour and sugar convert very rapidly, which causes a flood of glucose into your bloodstream. This "spike" of sugar in your blood requires a spike in insulin as well.

In the meantime your body works hard to maintain your blood sugar in a very specific range, but it's an imperfect process. Therefore, the spike in insulin is needed to quickly help deliver glucose to the cells and remove it from the blood. However, because of the rapid response from a large amount of insulin, blood sugar often drops too much.

The decrease in blood sugar can cause symptoms like fatigue, sugar cravings, headache, and irritability. This happens because your brain must have glucose to work properly. If the blood sugar is too low, you get dizzy, have headaches, and feel fatigue because your brain doesn't have adequate energy. You experience this as the crash after a sugar "high." As this spike and crash cycle continues, insulin becomes imbalanced and, as you will see, leads to a wide variety of other hormone imbalances.

Exactly what does it mean when your body doesn't "listen" to insulin well? The answer to this question can be found by comparing insulin to a pizza delivery man. In this analogy, insulin is a pizza delivery man and glucose, or sugar, is the pizza. A muscle cell is the house whose inhabitants have ordered a pizza. In the normal situation, when the people in the muscle cell house get hungry, they call out for a pizza. The pizza delivery man (insulin) picks up the pizza (glucose) and delivers it to the muscle cell house. He rings the doorbell to let them know that he is there; someone in the house opens the door; and the delivery man hands the pizza to him. This process seems fairly straightforward, doesn't it? Well, it works only when insulin is balanced.

Let's call the owner of the body George. In George's body are millions of muscle cells and millions of other types of cells as well. If year after year George eats a lot of refined carbohydrates such as white flour and sugars, he takes in a lot of sugar that creates thousands and thousands of pizzas (glucose) that need to be delivered.

Then George needs thousands and thousands of pizza delivery men (insulin). Imagine the scene now. The muscle cell neighborhood is swarming with delivery men who keep ringing the doorbells of the houses even if they have not ordered a pizza. Everyone in the muscle cell houses is overwhelmed. Every time the door of the house is opened, the muscle houses are assaulted by delivery men trying to get pizza into the house.

Remember, the job of the pizza delivery man (insulin) is to deliver pizza (glucose) no matter what because it's very dangerous to have extra glucose in the bloodstream. Eventually, the people in the muscle cell house are so overwhelmed, they close the shutters, lock the doors, stop answering the doorbell, and retreat to the center of the house. In medical terms, that is called *down regulating* your receptors. When you down regulate your receptors to any hormone, your cells stop listening to that hormone.

DEFINITION

Down regulating receptors are cells that allow hormones to communicate with the outside world. When there are too many hormones around the cell, it gets overwhelmed, pulls its receptors back inside, and stops communicating.

So now, the delivery men are left with many pizzas to deliver and no one in the muscle cell neighborhood willing to take them in. To solve this problem, they move over to the fat cell neighborhood. The people in the fat cell houses answer the doors when insulin knocks. They're friendlier because they can afford to be. They have a much higher capacity for taking the pizza in and storing it as fat.

Eventually, the pizza delivery men give up on the muscle cell neighborhood completely and go right to the fat cell neighborhood. When this happens, the vast majority of the sugar George eats ends up getting stored as fat.

As if having a lot of added fat wasn't bad enough, fat cells break down into cholesterol and triglycerides. So, as your muscle cells stop listening to insulin and shift to storing glucose in fat cells, the result is an increase in cholesterol and triglycerides. It's easy to see why a low-fat, low-cholesterol diet will not work to reduce heart disease, because the real culprit is glucose!

As you will see throughout this book, you can attack an insulin resistance problem a number of ways. First, you can stop eating foods that raise blood sugar and cause an increased demand for insulin. As fewer and fewer delivery men are running through the muscle cell neighborhoods, the muscle cells will eventually start answering their doors again. In medical terms, it means the cells up regulate their receptors and become sensitive to insulin again.

Another way you can work to reduce insulin resistance is to build lean muscle mass using strength training exercises. If you consider the analogy again, building new muscle cell houses in the neighborhood will not only give the delivery men more places to deliver pizza, but the people in the new houses won't know about the previous situation, so they will open the door for the delivery men. In this case, the new muscle cells are insulin sensitive, not insulin resistant.

The Food Guide Pyramid of the 1990s

In his book *Good Calories, Bad Calories*, Gary Taubes writes an extensive review of how low-fat, low-cholesterol foods became the nutritional gold standard in the United States in the 1990s. It was proclaimed to be the best way to prevent heart disease, and debates have raged through the '60s, '70s, and '80s, since science has never confirmed the benefits of this dietary approach.

A pivotal point in the entrenchment of this policy occurred in January of 1977, when Senator George McGovern published the first Dietary Goals for the United States. This was the first time a government institution (as opposed to private groups like the American Heart Association) told Americans they could improve their health by eating less fat. The government publication of Dietary Goals sparked a chain reaction of dietary advice from government agencies and the media that continues to this day.

Taubes notes that the publication of Dietary Goals changed a lot about how Americans get their health recommendations. The most interesting thing about the low-fat, low-cholesterol concept is that there has not been a lot of data to support it. Taubes writes, "Dietary Goals took a grab bag of ambiguous studies and speculation, acknowledged that the claims were scientifically contentious and then officially bestowed on one interpretation the aura of established fact." The Dietary Goals document was written by Senator McGovern's staff who were not scientists and were virtually unaware of the existence of any scientific controversy. The fact that it came from the government created the illusion that the science was sound.

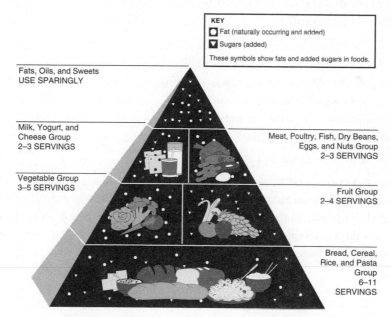

The 1992 Food Guide Pyramid.
(Courtesy of the U.S. Department of Agriculture)

One problem with the government giving health-care information is that government policy is often tied to industry. For example, the Food Guide Pyramid of 1992 was developed by the U.S. Department of Agriculture (USDA), whose mission is to promote and support agriculture. The pyramid recommended 6 to 11 servings of bread, cereal, rice, and pasta. It also told us to "use fat sparingly," but did not define exactly what "sparingly" was. Because of the way hormones like insulin work and how closely insulin is connected to other hormones, this diet has been a recipe for disaster.

To make matters worse, the Food Guide Pyramid became the basis of school lunch programs, hospital food programs, nursing-home menus, and all federally funded institutions that serve food.

THAT'S QUOTABLE

"The [1992] pyramid is really not compatible with good scientific evidence, and it was really out of date from the day it was printed in 1991."

—Walter Willett, Chair, Nutrition Department, Harvard School of Public Health

Because of government policy, in the 1980s and 1990s, we all thought we were doing the right thing by buying and eating "fat-free" this and "low-cholesterol" that. And we now had permission to eat lots of bagels, cereals, and pasta! The result was that many of us slowly became insulin resistant, a condition in which our muscle cells stop listening to insulin, and we preferentially store our sugar as fat.

So we packed on the pounds. We struggled to reduce our fat intake even further and stopped eating anything with cholesterol—eggs, shrimp, and shellfish. To our surprise, the weight continued to creep up, and so did our cholesterol. Some of us tried exercising as often as possible. Yet the weight wouldn't budge and, on top of that, we were tired, our skin was dry, and it became harder to concentrate. Oh yes, and our sex drives existed only in our memories.

The truth is that our bodies need fat in order to function. As a matter of fact, the majority of our brain is made up of fat. (So, we are all fatheads!) The sooner we appreciate the way our bodies work and we get away from the low-fat, low-cholesterol shackles, the faster we can balance our hormones, feel better, and maintain our optimal weight.

The Least You Need to Know

- Obesity is on the rise, and dieting isn't taking care of the problem.
- Among others, processed foods, high fructose corn syrup, and toxins lead to weight gain.
- Insulin resistance causes most of the sugar you eat to be stored as fat.
- Government recommendations to eat low-fat, low-cholesterol foods have not helped to prevent heart disease and have caused many of us to gain weight.

The Power of Hormones

In This Chapter

- The importance of hormone balance
- Steroid hormones: the good news about cholesterol
- Hormone pathways
- Stress, toxins, and weight gain

We very rarely pay attention to the importance of hormones in our lives. However, we all depend on them for survival and well-being every minute of every day. This chapter looks at the power that hormones have over your body.

Hormones: A Balancing Act

In their role as chemical messengers, hormones help determine your mood, energy level, ability to concentrate, weight, and many other things. They also help your body maintain all of its functions such as your temperature, pulse, metabolism, immune function, appetite, libido, and even your ability to form memories.

What are these powerful messengers? Hormones are chemicals that flow through your bloodstream to deliver information from one set of cells to another. They are produced in your endocrine glands, which secrete them directly into your circulation or ducts. In addition, men and women produce hormones in their reproductive organs.

Hormones are potent. Very small amounts can pack a wallop. And too much, too little, or an alteration of a hormone's structure can upset your *metabolism* and cause you to gain weight.

DEFINITION

Metabolism is the process of turning digested food, stored fat, or muscle into calories that the body uses as energy.

Hormones deliver their messages by communicating with your body's cells through connections called receptors. Hormone receptors are proteins that are embedded in the outside walls of cells. They work like locks and keys. Each hormone—whether estrogen, cortisol, or another type of hormone—connects only with the cells that it's programmed by nature to match. The reverse is also true. Each cell in your body has many receptors that are designed to join only with the hormones or molecules that are specific to them. Any changes to the structure or shape of the hormones make it difficult for receptors to connect. It's like a key with an extra prong; it doesn't work as well in the lock.

In this complex system, a number of scenarios can occur that may result in your body not getting the right amount of hormone activity it needs:

- On the one hand, you may have enough receptors on a cell but have the wrong type of hormone, so you don't get the responses from the cells that you need.

- On the other hand, sometimes a cell reduces the number of receptors it has, so even if you have enough of the matching hormone, the cell isn't "listening."

A cell can also voluntarily reduce the number of available receptors it has for a particular hormone, in which case it's said to have "resistance" to that hormone. Take insulin resistance as an example. If you consume a diet high in sugars and refined carbohydrates for a long time, you will need a lot of the hormone insulin to remove the sugar from your blood. If cells are exposed to large amounts of insulin for a long time, the cells, in order to protect themselves from too much of the hormone, pull their receptors inside and shut down for business. The result is that your body acts like it doesn't have enough insulin.

DID YOU KNOW?

Insulin resistance can be deceiving. For example, if at the point just described, we take a sample of your blood and look at the amount of insulin available, there would probably be more than enough insulin. But the cells pulled back their receptors, so they're not listening to it. Subsequently, your blood sugar might also be high, which is one way that your doctor would know you are insulin resistant—there's enough insulin, but it's not doing its job.

Hormones in Harmony

Hormones function best when, like the instruments in a well-tuned orchestra, they are correctly balanced. If any instrument is missing, overpowering, or out of tune, it can throw off an entire performance.

The good news is that your body has an elegant system to maintain the balance among its hormones. Your brain constantly samples different areas of your body to make sure its hormone levels are in the correct range. If your levels are too high, your brain sends a message to the appropriate gland to reduce production. If your levels are too low, your brain signals the gland to increase production.

Unfortunately, many things can upset this balance system, including stress, poor diet, food allergies, toxins, and the environment.

Steroids

Steroid hormones are important pieces of the metabolism puzzle. You need to understand the following basic points about hormones:

- *Cortisol*, also known as the "fight or flight" hormone, is one of your stress hormones. Along with adrenaline, its main function is to help you handle emergencies that occur, real or imagined, inside or outside of your body. Two main hormone building blocks, *pregnenolone* and *progesterone*, produce cortisol and come directly from cholesterol.

- Although both men and women have it, *testosterone* is known as the "male sex hormone." Among other things, the hormone helps build bones and lean muscle mass, which creates energy and keeps weight down.

- *Estrogen*, known as the "female sex hormone," is also found in men and women and has more than 400 functions in the body, including increasing metabolism, which controls weight.

- *DHEA* is a hormone that helps build muscle and bone and helps make insulin work better, both of which affect weight.

Cholesterol

Many people are afraid of *cholesterol* because they associate it with heart disease. However, in the face of extensive campaigns for Americans to eat low-fat, low-cholesterol diets, rates of heart disease remain high.

DEFINITION

Cholesterol is a waxy substance produced in our bodies and found in our diets. It's an essential part of cell membranes; bile acids; steroid hormones; and the fat-soluble vitamins A, E, D, and K. The typical body normally produces about 1,000 milligrams per day.

The reality is that a low-fat, low-cholesterol diet usually contains a lot of sugar to compensate for the flavor lost by the reduction in fat. Because of insulin resistance, much of this sugar ends up being stored as fat. The increase in stored fat causes a release of cholesterol and triglycerides, which are markers for heart disease, into the blood. Therefore, it is actually excess sugar, not excess cholesterol, that causes an increase in blood cholesterol.

It's important to know that cholesterol serves many important purposes in your body and is critical for the production of steroid hormones. As a matter of fact, if your total cholesterol level is too low, you may not be making enough hormones! And if you consistently have high cholesterol despite appropriate diet and lifestyle, it may be a sign of hormone imbalance because your body is trying to make enough extra cholesterol to produce hormones.

Hormone Building Blocks

The hormones pregnenolone and progesterone come directly from cholesterol and are the building blocks for all other steroid hormones. Depending on the needs of the body, they produce two major groups of hormones:

- The stress hormone cortisol (pathway 1)

- The sex hormones DHEA, estrogen, and testosterone (pathway 2)

Remember this important fact: the building block hormones pregnenolone and progesterone have a choice in which pathway they follow. They can either follow pathway 1 and produce cortisol or follow pathway 2 to produce DHEA, estrogen, and testosterone. This fact is important when you look at how your stress levels and toxins influence your hormone levels. If you constantly have a high stress level, you will have a high demand for cortisol. Subsequently, your building blocks will preferentially follow pathway 1 to make cortisol and you will make less DHEA, testosterone, and estrogen.

Stress and Demands on Your Hormones

Most people think of stress as emotional tension or feeling overwhelmed. However, a lot of other stressors continually bombard people, such as infections, food allergies, low blood sugar, heat or cold, and lack of sleep.

Cortisol is one of the hormones that enables the human body to handle these stressors. The catch is that because it's designed for short-term, intense crises, the role it plays works well for emergencies (such as running from a burning building) but not everyday stresses (such as screaming bosses or stretched finances).

In Chapter 1, you learned about high blood sugar, insulin resistance, and the reasons we store extra sugar as fat. High cortisol increases blood sugar, and stress of any type increases the demand for cortisol. Therefore, chronic increased stress leads to increases in blood sugar and subsequent insulin resistance. This leads to more fat storage, weight gain, and … well, you get the picture.

The Cortisol Response

Think back to the time of cavemen. One of their major stressors was the real possibility of being attacked by saber-toothed tigers. Then think about all the things that have to happen in your body to outrun such a beast. This gives you an idea of what the cortisol response to stress does to your body.

In order to run, your circulatory system needs to send a lot of blood to your muscles to give them oxygen. As a result, your intestines will have less blood than they normally do, and you will not be able to digest food well.

Your body also needs to get a lot of sugar into your bloodstream to give energy to your muscles. In addition, your blood pressure must go up, your awareness of pain must go down, and your blood clotting factors must increase in case you're injured during the chase. And while all this is happening, your body will do all it can to slow down your metabolism so you can save enough energy to handle stress when you most need it.

Long-Term Stress

The cortisol response was meant to be short-lived. (If you outran the tiger, you didn't need any more of it, and if you were eaten by the tiger, you didn't need it anymore.) Today, people are under great, long-term stress and have a constant high demand for cortisol. For many, the constant bombarding of cortisol has negative, long-term consequences.

One consequence of cortisol overload is that it keeps your body from making adequate amounts of your most active thyroid hormone, T3 or triiodothyronine (one of four types of thyroid hormones). In effect, this slows down your metabolism, which is helpful if you're being chased by that tiger or have a very low food supply due to famine. A similar situation can occur after a "crash diet," when you have significantly restricted your calories. Here's what happens: your body thinks there is a famine; your cortisol level goes up; your thyroid function goes down; and not only does your weight loss slow, but once you start eating a regular diet, you gain weight much more quickly.

However, if your stress comes from taxes, your boss, or your relationships, a low metabolism can actually be harmful because you're not doing anything extra to burn energy, and you need fewer calories to survive. If you don't adjust your diet to eat fewer calories, you will gain weight.

THAT'S QUOTABLE

"Our modern diet screwed up all the hormones that play a role in weight and health. Our ancestors did not consume soda, sweets, cereals, fat-free food, skim milk, refined vegetable oils, margarine, artificial sweeteners, or alcohol. Much of this food was never meant for human consumption, and we moved from a hormone-friendly diet to a hormone unfriendly diet."

—Michael Aziz, M.D., *The Perfect 10 Diet,* Sourcebooks, 2010

Stress and the Sex Hormones

Remember that the building blocks for cortisol, pregnenolone, and progesterone are the same building blocks as those for your sex hormones, estrogen and testosterone. Therefore, if your stress levels remain high, your supply of building blocks will be focused on producing stress hormones (pathway 1) and may be too low to make enough sex hormones (pathway 2).

This imbalance can cause havoc in your body and promote weight gain because testosterone helps you to build lean muscle mass, which helps you burn up more energy and increase your metabolism. Estrogen is also known to help increase metabolism. If their production is reduced, you will burn less energy and gain weight.

Progesterone, one of the building blocks, is also important in balancing estrogen levels in the body. If estrogen and progesterone are not well balanced and your metabolism is decreased, symptoms such as weight gain, mood changes, sleep disturbances, and water retention can occur.

Are You Building Up or Breaking Down?

Bodies are changing constantly. Even the parts that seem stable, like bones, are continually evolving. Hormones play an important role in this process. They break down (*catabolic*) or build up (*anabolic*) tissues in the body. The hormone cortisol breaks down body tissues such as fat and muscle and "harvests" its energy-producing building blocks. These building blocks are made into sugar, which end up in the bloodstream.

DEFINITION

Catabolic are pathways that break down molecules into smaller units and release energy.

Anabolic are metabolic pathways that construct molecules from smaller units; these reactions require energy.

Extra Blood Sugar

Extra blood sugar is helpful if your muscles need energy to fight or flee. However, many of the current stressors, such as emotional stress or lack of sleep, don't require extra blood sugar for energy. The result is the breakdown of healthy muscle tissue and an overload of blood sugar. Over a period of time, this creates problems with insulin resistance and contributes to further weight gain.

Reduced Sex Hormones and Increased Belly Fat

Sex hormones have a role that is the opposite of cortisol. They help build and repair the body. Estrogen, progesterone, and testosterone all support healthy bone growth. As described earlier, testosterone supports the growth of lean muscle mass and reduces fat mass. It's easy to see how an imbalance in these hormones creates an unhealthy metabolism and an overload of sugar in the blood.

And there's even more bad news. High cortisol levels cause an increase in the production of belly fat, which leads to weight gain and inflammation. Scientists have taken a special interest in belly fat, which is very different from the fat in other parts of your body. One of the problems with belly fat, in addition to being unsightly, is that it's actually its own endocrine organ! It can produce hormones and inflammatory molecules, and it has enzymes in it that turn testosterone into estrogen. In small amounts, this is a good thing. However, if there is a lot of belly fat and the majority of testosterone is being turned into estrogen in men or women, the result is reduction in the amount of lean muscle mass created, which contributes to weight gain.

Belly fat is inflammatory, which means that it creates irritation in the body and makes people more likely to develop arthritis, allergies, or other problems. The combination of belly fat and inflammation can act as another stressor, setting off another vicious circle because the inflammation creates even more of a demand for cortisol, which leads to more belly fat and then to more inflammation.

TRUSTY TIP

Read *The Complete Idiot's Guide to Inflammation* and *The Complete Idiot's Guide to the Anti-Inflammation Diet* for tips to help you reduce your level of inflammation and cortisol demand.

Cortisol and the Thyroid

Keep in mind that high cortisol levels also affect the function of the thyroid gland, the master of the metabolism. Our thyroid gland is located in our lower neck and produces a few different types of thyroid hormone. For this explanation, we focus on two of them: thyroxine (T4) and triiodothyronine (T3). Our thyroid gland produces mainly T4, which has some activity. However, we rely on our body to turn T4 into T3 outside of the thyroid gland, and T3 has five times as much activity as T4. So for a healthy metabolism, you need to convert T4 to T3.

The production of the most active thyroid hormone, T3, is inhibited by high cortisol levels. Therefore, the more stress a person has, the lower her metabolism, the fewer calories she burns, and the heavier she becomes. In addition, low thyroid hormone causes a number of other problems such as difficulty concentrating, dry skin, constipation, and fatigue. So the higher the stress level, the more likely you are to suffer from a number of symptoms besides weight gain.

Toxins and Hormone Imbalance

Not only do bodies produce hormones based on what happens inside, they also make them in reaction to what happens outside the body. And if a lot of toxins are in the environment, the result is a faulty production or use of hormones that leads to an imbalance.

You should be concerned about three major types of toxins: pesticides, *Bisphenol A (BPA)*, and *phthalates*. These three substances are known as "endocrine disrupters," because they can change the way the body produces hormones and how hormones interact within the body. Evidence of the link between toxins and obesity is so strong that a new term has sprung up to describe these substances: *obesegens*.

Bisphenol A (BPA) is a chemical produced in large quantities for use primarily in the production of polycarbonate plastics and epoxy resins. It's a known endocrine disruptor.

Phthalates are eaters of phthalic acid and are mainly used as plasticizers (substances added to plastics to increase their flexibility, transparency, durability, and longevity). Phthalates are known endocrine disruptors.

Obesegens are chemicals that scientists believe promote weight gain and obesity. They may do this by increasing the number of fat cells, reducing the number of calories burned at rest, altering energy balance, or changing your mechanisms for appetite and satiety.

As endocrine disrupters, pesticides, phthalates, and BPA can affect estrogen and thyroid hormone. When thyroid hormone is interfered with, your metabolism goes down and you burn fewer calories, making it easier to gain weight.

Also, these toxins create inflammation and irritation in your body, which increases cortisol demand and leads to further hormone imbalance and weight gain.

Pesticides

Pesticide is a global term for any substance that destroys insects and other unwanted pests such as mice, roaches, and weeds. Pesticides are also used to destroy organisms that we don't usually think of as pests but are potentially harmful to humans such as fungi, bacteria, and viruses. Many household products are pesticides, including cockroach sprays and baits; kitchen, laundry, and bath disinfectants and sanitizers; and lawn and garden products.

Bisphenol A

Bisphenol A (BPA) is an organic compound used to make plastics and resins. High levels of BPA are associated with obesity, insulin resistance, and thyroid problems. BPA is found in plastic water bottles, baby bottles, and the lining of aluminum cans. It often finds its way into what people eat and drink. For example, a recent Health Canada study found that the majority of canned soft drinks it tested had measurable amounts of BPA. In September 2010, Canada became the first country to officially declare BPA a toxic substance.

Phthalates

Phthalates are substances that are added to plastics to increase their flexibility, transparency, durability, and longevity. Phthalates are found in flexible plastics and many hair care, home care, and skin care products. We discuss them in much greater detail in Chapter 4.

Toxins are not easy to avoid. They are in foods, drinks, baby formulas, water bottles, hair and skin care products, and many other things you come in contact with every day. The good news is that your liver is good at removing these toxins. If exposure to them is limited, your hormones will be more balanced and your weight will be more under control.

The Least You Need to Know

- A correct hormone balance is necessary to maintain a healthy weight.
- In order for your body to produce hormones, it has to have adequate supplies of cholesterol.
- An imbalance in sex and stress hormones creates an unhealthy metabolism and an overload of blood sugar.
- Stress leads to high cortisol levels, which increases belly fat and causes weight gain.
- Toxins can also cause a hormone imbalance.

How Hormones Can Make You Fat

In This Chapter

- The key hormones related to weight and how they work
- How our bodies develop resistance and fail to respond to hormones
- The vicious cycle of hormone imbalance and fat storage

The human body has more than 100 hormones. Some have a limited function, and others are key to survival. Understanding how hormones work can help you make healthy choices. A problem with any of the 10 hormones discussed in this chapter can result in weight gain and difficulties in losing weight.

This chapter describes the hormones that are related to weight and what each one does. It also lists symptoms of hormone imbalance and the causes and conditions related to imbalance.

Insulin

Insulin is probably the most important hormone produced when it comes to maintaining a healthy weight. It originates in the beta cells of the pancreas. Although insulin plays a role in numerous functions in the body, its most important function is to stabilize blood sugar levels. If your level of glucose is too high, it can cause damage to your smallest blood vessels, especially those in your eyes and kidneys. This is why people with long-standing diabetes or high blood sugar tend to have problems with blindness and kidney disease. On the other hand, if your blood glucose level is too low, your cells, especially the cells in your brain that run mainly on glucose, will not have enough energy (which can lead to death).

Insulin and Diet

Insulin resistance causes high blood sugar, diabetes, and other health problems. To reduce your risk of insulin resistance, follow the diet plan in Chapters 20 and 21. This plan promotes foods that are low in sugars and refined carbohydrates and high in vegetables, high-fiber fruits, lean proteins, and healthy fats.

Symptoms and Causes of Insulin Problems

The following list includes symptoms of insulin resistance, causes of insulin imbalance, and symptoms of insulin deficiency. If you have two or more of these symptoms, you should discuss them with your doctor.

Symptoms of insulin resistance (too much insulin) include:

- Abdominal obesity (waist > 40 inches for men; waist > 35 inches for women)
- Acanthosis nigricans (dark spots on elbows, armpits, neck, and groin)
- Decreased memory or concentration
- Elevated fasting blood sugar (> 100 mg/dL; identified by blood tests)
- Elevated liver enzymes (identified by blood tests)
- Elevated triglycerides (identified by blood tests)
- Irregular bowel movements (diarrhea alternating with constipation)
- Irregular menstrual periods

Other symptoms include acne, ankle swelling, constipation, depression, fatigue, gout, high blood pressure, infertility, a low libido, skin tags, water retention, and weight gain.

Causes of insulin imbalance (too much insulin) include:

- Alcohol abuse
- Birth control pills (or other progestins)
- Chronic elevated stress
- Decreased estrogen (female) or decreased testosterone (male)
- Excess DHEA, dieting, caffeine intake, or progesterone (female)
- Hypothyroidism

- Infections

- Insomnia

- Lack of exercise

- Nicotine (smoking)

- Obesity

- Skipping breakfast (and other meals)

Symptoms of insulin deficiency (not enough insulin) include:

- Blurred vision and/or dizziness

- Excessive thirst and/or increased urination

- Fatigue

- Infections

- Rapid breathing and/or rapid heart rate

- Vomiting

- Weight loss

Cortisol

Cortisol is the second most important hormone when it comes to weight gain. It's often referred to as the "stress hormone." It comes from the adrenal cortex, which is the outer part of the adrenal gland located on top of the kidney. Cortisol is released as a response to stress and anxiety. It has three major functions that allow you to handle stressors: it increases blood sugar levels (increases available energy to deal with the stress), raises blood pressure, and reduces inflammation.

TRUSTY TIP

Some stress can be good. Many world-class athletes use their stress in a productive way to get "in the zone," in which the extreme stress and high cortisol allows them to increase their ability to focus and concentrate. They use the extra energy they have available to them through stress to excel in their sports.

Cortisol is a catabolic, or breakdown, hormone. For there to be a large release of energy when you're under stress, cortisol directs the breakdown of the various tissues such as fat, muscle, and bone.

Initially, it sounds good that cortisol breaks down fat. However, it tends to break down more important tissues like muscle and bone even more. Also, since one of cortisol's jobs is to replace the energy that was used in the initial response to stress, cortisol increases your appetite and makes you crave high-carbohydrate, high-fat foods.

When cortisol is elevated for a long period of time, it stimulates the deposit of a specific kind of fat called *visceral fat*. Visceral fat is found around your organs and is the source of fat around your stomach.

Most people are surprised to find out that visceral fat is an endocrine organ and has enzymes that affect other hormone levels such as estrogen and testosterone. In addition, it secretes molecules called *cytokines* that increase inflammation in the body. Since one of the jobs of cortisol is to reduce inflammation, you can see that you get into another vicious cycle that goes like this: Increased cortisol causes increased belly fat, which leads to increased cytokine production and inflammation. This leads to increased cortisol production, which leads to even more belly fat.

High cortisol also increases the chance that you will develop a food addiction, which happens because your brain releases chemicals called *endorphins* that make you feel good whenever you eat (especially when you consume carbohydrates). So when you feel stressed, your cortisol level goes up; you crave high-fat, high-carbohydrate foods; you eat those foods; and your brain releases endorphins that make you feel better. Eventually, you associate eating when stressed with feeling better and can become mentally and physically dependent on eating as a way to manage stress. This vicious cycle can become entrenched.

DEFINITION

Visceral fat is found around your organs. You need some visceral fat to protect your organs. However, it is very inflammatory and is the source of the fat around our midsections (belly fat).

Cytokines are proteins that serve as messengers between cells and regulate inflammatory responses.

Endorphins are chemicals produced by the body that suppress pain and make you feel good.

If you have long-term stress in your life and your cortisol levels remain high, you might get to a point at which your body starts to resist weight loss. Why does this happen? The main chronic stressor for early humans was famine. So your body naturally thinks that when you're in a chronic stress situation, it must be a famine and foods must not be available. Therefore, it tries to store any food that you eat and hold on to any fat that you already have. High cortisol levels cause a reduction in the levels of your most active thyroid hormone, which greatly reduces your metabolism. So you continue to store belly fat and can't break down any other fat you have in your body.

In addition, adrenal fatigue can occur after a period of prolonged stress. The result is that your adrenal glands can no longer supply enough cortisol to meet your demands. It's important to understand that weight loss is extremely difficult with too much or too little cortisol.

TRUSTY TIP

If you suspect your cortisol levels are too high or too low, have your hormone levels tested. The good news is that by following the seven principles of the diet plan outlined in Part 2, you will balance your cortisol and begin to heal your metabolism.

The long-term effects of high cortisol include:

- Belly fat
- Binge eating
- Confusion, depression, and/or irritability
- Decreased immune response
- Diabetes
- Easily bruising
- Fatigue and/or insomnia
- Frequent colds or infections
- High blood pressure and/or high blood sugar
- High cholesterol and triglycerides
- Increased osteoporosis risk
- Insulin resistance
- Irregular periods
- Low libido
- Muscle weakness
- Sugar cravings and/or weight gain

Conditions associated with abnormal cortisol levels include:

- Addison's disease, anorexia nervosa, chronic fatigue syndrome, Cushing's syndrome, panic disorders, and adrenal insufficiency
- Depression
- Diabetes, fibromyalgia, osteoporosis, and heart disease
- Impotence and infertility
- Insomnia
- Menopause/andropause and PMS

Symptoms of cortisol deficiency (adrenal fatigue) include:

- Alcohol and drug addiction and chemical intolerance
- Allergies
- Apathy, emotional liability, and loss of motivation
- Extreme weakness and chronic fatigue
- Increased PMS/menopausal/ andropause symptoms

- Low blood pressure
- Low sex drive
- Nervousness/irritability
- Recurrent respiratory infections
- Salt cravings
- Slow recovery from trauma or illness
- Unresponsive hypothyroidism

Causes of cortisol imbalance include:

- Allergies
- Chronic stress
- Depression, frustration, anger, loss of control, and unpredictability
- Excessive caffeine and sugar
- Insomnia/poor sleep habits

- Irregular eating habits/skipping breakfast
- Novelty
- Obesity
- Toxin exposure

Glucagon

Glucagon, like insulin, is produced in the pancreas. It counterbalances insulin. The job of insulin is to help nutrients get into the cells, and the job of glucagon is to release those stored nutrients to be used for energy as needed. Insulin and glucagon have complementary roles in allowing you to have the right energy levels for your body at all times.

Glucagon promotes the release of stored glucose (known as glycogen) from the liver and the release of free fatty acids from your fat stores. Therefore, this hormone actually helps you break down fat. Because glucagon is a counterbalancing hormone to insulin, they aren't present at the same time. The pancreas is either releasing insulin in response to sugar or releasing glucagon in response to protein foods. Neither insulin nor glucagon is released when nonstarchy vegetables and fats are consumed.

As insulin lets nutrients such as amino acids and sugar into cells, it achieves two major goals. First, the body is replenished and renewed, and blood sugar levels are balanced. Second, insulin tells the liver when too much sugar has entered, and the liver reacts by increasing fat production from the incoming sugar. The ratio between insulin and glucagon determines whether food is used as building materials and fuel or stored as fat. A higher proportion of glucagon means that more food is used as building material or fuel.

A high-carbohydrate diet causes problems with levels of glucagon. Due to this kind of diet, many people overproduce insulin and don't produce enough glucagon. You can heal your metabolism and encourage glucagon to burn fat by balancing your insulin. When you eat natural fats and adequate amounts of protein, eliminate refined carbohydrates, and exercise, you naturally increase your levels of glucagon, which encourages your body to use nutrients as fuel and building blocks for muscle and other important tissues in your body and to not store them as fat.

The following are factors that affect the level of glucagon in the body. Factors that increase glucagon include:

- Diet low in sugar and low blood sugar
- Exercise
- Increased blood amino acid levels (eating protein)
- Protein foods
- Skipping meals and/or starvation (not recommended)

Factors that decrease glucagon include:

- Free fatty acids in the blood (from too much sugar)
- Frequent meals
- High blood sugar
- Insulin
- Refined carbohydrates in diet
- Sedentary lifestyle

Leptin

Leptin regulates appetites and metabolisms. The hormone was discovered in 1995 and thought to be a major key to weight loss. Leptin manages how much fat is stored around your organs and under your skin by acting on receptors in the brain and throughout your body.

Leptin is secreted by fat cells to indicate that the body has had enough food. When the fat cells are filled with food, they secrete leptin. The leptin travels to your hypothalamus, which is the part of your brain that controls your appetite, and attaches to the leptin receptors. These receptors increase or decrease the production of *neuropeptides*, chemical messengers that help to turn your appetite on and off. Leptin acts by turning *neuropeptide Y* off so your body turns down its appetite and turns up its metabolism. If this intricate system is working the right way, when you've had enough to eat, your fat cells secrete leptin; the leptin goes to your brain to curb your appetite; and, as a result, you feel satisfied.

DEFINITION

Neuropeptides are chemicals similar to proteins that are released by neurons (brain cells) to carry messages between cells.

Neuropeptide Y is the most abundant neuropeptide in the brain. It stimulates hunger.

Initially, scientists thought that if they gave leptin to overweight people, their appetite would go down and they would burn more fat. However, they tried it to no avail. As a matter of fact, when they measured leptin levels in overweight people, they found that they had too much leptin! This happens because refined carbohydrates, trans fats, and elevated insulin levels are associated with higher leptin levels. Elevated insulin levels and diets high in refined carbohydrates cause excess fat storage in the body. Because these foods are so low in nutritional value, the body actually thinks it's starving. It doesn't have the right nutrients and sends signals to the brain to make the body burn fewer calories and store fat even in the presence of high leptin levels.

If you're overweight, you can develop resistance to leptin in the same way that you can develop insulin resistance. The receptors on your cells become so overwhelmed by high levels of leptin, they eventually stop listening to it. Because they are not responding to leptin, your body acts like you have low levels of leptin and feels hungry most of the time. In this case, the cells don't turn off neuropeptide Y, you remain hungry even if you ate, and your metabolism remains slow.

High leptin levels and leptin resistance can be a problem as you try to lose weight. However, you can break the cycle that causes leptin resistance and help your cells to start listening to the hormone again. The best way to do this is by eating foods that do not contain refined carbohydrates, trans fats, artificial sweeteners, and high fructose corn syrup. Focus on vegetables, fruits, proteins, and natural fats. (In other words, follow the hormone weight-loss diet!)

The following consist of factors that disturb leptin levels and symptoms of leptin resistance and leptin deficiency. Symptoms of too much leptin (leptin resistance) include:

- Diabetes and heart disease
- High blood pressure and high cholesterol
- Hunger (unable to satisfy)
- Inflammation
- Insulin resistance
- Obesity

Symptoms of too little leptin include:

- Anorexia nervosa
- Depression
- Hunger (unable to satisfy)

Things that disturb leptin include:

- Aging
- Belly fat (abdominal obesity)
- High fructose corn syrup
- Infection
- Inflammation
- Insomnia (less than seven to eight hours of sleep per night)
- Menopause
- Obesity
- Pain
- Refined carbohydrates
- Smoking
- Stress
- Trans fats

Ghrelin

Ghrelin is a hormone that balances leptin. Leptin tells the brain that you're satisfied and turns off hunger; ghrelin tells the brain that you're hungry. In addition to stimulating hunger and increasing food intake, it also increases the amount of fat in your body. Ghrelin also helps to stimulate the secretion of growth hormone.

Ghrelin comes from cells in the lining of the stomach, duodenum, and upper intestine. It's also produced by the epsilon cells of the pancreas and hypothalamus where it stimulates the secretion of growth hormone.

The main function of ghrelin is to increase hunger. The levels of ghrelin go up when your stomach is empty and will stay up until your body has enough nutrients to be satisfied. As your stomach fills, the levels of ghrelin start to drop, you feel satisfied, and your hunger decreases. Like leptin, ghrelin does its work by acting on the signaling protein, neuropeptide Y. However, instead of turning it off like leptin, ghrelin turns it on. Remember, neuropeptide Y acts to increase your hunger and slow down your metabolism, so you don't want too much of this hanging around!

Another function of ghrelin is to get you through the four stages of sleep. During stage IV, the deepest stage, which usually occurs during the first 90 minutes of your sleep, ghrelin stimulates the release of growth hormone. Growth hormone is a master hormone that helps build muscle and burn fat. You definitely want to have good levels of this hormone! Also, leptin is secreted so that you don't wake up during the middle of the night to find something to eat. Before you go to sleep, you want your ghrelin levels to be high so you get through the stages of sleep. For that reason, it's best to stop eating a few hours before you go to sleep so that your ghrelin levels have a chance to rise. Interestingly, inadequate sleep is associated with high ghrelin levels. This is one of the reasons why sleep disturbance can lead to increased appetite and eating more food than your body uses.

Ghrelin can become imbalanced because of lack of sleep and frequent dieting. People with eating disorders often have significant imbalances. Those with anorexia nervosa tend to have much higher levels of ghrelin than most people. However, they are one of the few groups of people that may feel better with these higher levels. It may act as an antidepressant for them. The best way to keep ghrelin stable is to get adequate sleep and eat healthy, balanced meals every three to four hours.

Things that increase ghrelin include:

- Calorie restriction and skipping meals
- Hypothyroidism
- Inadequate protein and carbohydrate intake and high fat intake
- Insomnia/sleep disturbance
- Stress

Thyroid

The thyroid is one of the largest glands that produces hormones in the body. It's critical not only to your metabolism but as a regulator of numerous other functions in your body, including energy and heat production, tissue repair, regulating protein, carbohydrate and fat metabolism, and muscle and nerve action.

The thyroid gland is a butterfly-shaped gland located in the front portion of your neck. It's just under your thyroid cartilage (also known as the Adam's apple) and above your collarbone.

> **DID YOU KNOW?**
>
> The thyroid gland is the only gland that has the ability to store a hormone; it can store up to about 100 days' worth of hormone.

Your body produces more than one type of thyroid hormone. The main thyroid hormone is called thyroxine (T4); another hormone, triiodothyronine (T3), is produced in small amounts by the thyroid and converted from T4 in your liver and kidneys. This becomes very important because, since your thyroid releases mostly T4, you rely very heavily on the conversion from T4 to T3 in your body for an active metabolism. The conversion is important because T3 is five times more active than T4. If you don't convert enough T4 to T3, your metabolism is slower, and it's much harder to lose weight.

From aging to zinc deficiency, the following lists the large range of factors that can interfere with this conversion, lower your metabolism, and cause weight gain. Factors that reduce the conversion of T4 to T3 include:

- Aging
- Cadmium, mercury, or lead toxicity
- Calcium access
- Chronic illness
- Decreased liver kidney function
- Elevated cortisol
- Iodine deficiency and iron deficiency
- Low-fat diet, low-protein diet, and high-carbohydrate diet
- Medications (beta blockers, birth control pills, estrogen)
- Pesticides
- Phthalates
- Selenium and zinc deficiency
- Starvation/low-calorie diet

Your thyroid controls many things in your body, including digestion and the rate you burn calories. Therefore, if your thyroid becomes overactive or underactive, it affects many aspects of your body at the same time.

If your thyroid is underactive, or you are *hypothyroid*, the effects are far-reaching. You may feel sluggish, have difficulty concentrating, have difficulty losing weight, have cold hands or feet, and experience constipation, among other things. Hypothyroidism has a number of causes. The most common diagnosed cause is Hashimoto's thyroiditis, which is a disease of the body's immune system. If you have this condition, it means that your body makes *antibodies* against thyroid tissue, which makes it more difficult for you to produce enough hormone and for it to attach to your thyroid receptors. The result is that it's not able to do its job of regulating your metabolism, digestion, and other functions. Hashimoto's thyroiditis, like most *autoimmune* diseases, is much more common in women.

DEFINITION

Hypothyroid means that your thyroid is underactive.

Antibodies are proteins that the immune system uses to fight off offenders such as bacteria and viruses.

Autoimmune diseases are caused by the body making antibodies against normal tissue in the body (such as the thyroid), which creates damage to the tissue.

A strong connection also exists between thyroid antibodies and gluten sensitivity. Studies have shown that some women who are hypothyroid can return to normal thyroid function simply by removing gluten from their diet. Even if you still need thyroid replacement, removing gluten from your diet can make your thyroid function and hormone balance even better.

If your thyroid hormone production is low (the symptoms of which are detailed in the following list), or the rate that you convert T4 to T3 is low, you may have symptoms of hypothyroidism. Because thyroid hormone is used in so many places in the body, the symptoms can be quite varied and extensive. In Chapter 15, I discuss hormone testing at length. If you think that you have symptoms of low thyroid, talk to your physician about thyroid testing.

Symptoms of low thyroid production (hypothyroidism) include:

- Anxiety, depression, and difficulty concentrating
- Cold intolerance—cold hands and feet
- Dry hair and skin; brittle nails; hair loss; hoarse voice; puffy face; and swollen legs, feet, and hands
- Fatigue and/or insomnia

- Fluid retention and constipation
- Irregular, heavy menses

- Muscle pain and cramping
- Weight gain

On the opposite end of the spectrum, Graves' disease, or *hyperthyroidism*, is an auto-immune disease in which the thyroid is overactive. Graves' is the most common cause of hyperthyroidism and can create a lot of uncomfortable symptoms such as heart palpitations, heat intolerance, severe weight loss, diarrhea, dizziness, and bulging eyes. It can be dangerous, and patients with this condition need to be watched very closely by an endocrinologist (a doctor who specializes in hormones). People with Graves' disease may need to take medication to block their overactive thyroid. In severe cases, they may need to have their thyroid destroyed with radioactive iodine. If their thyroid is destroyed, they become hypothyroid and will need thyroid replacement.

DEFINITION

Hyperthyroid means that your thyroid is overactive.

Symptoms of high thyroid production (hyperthyroidism) include:

- Diarrhea
- Dizziness, heat intolerance, rapid pulse, and sweating
- Exophthalmus (bulging eyes)
- Fatigue and insomnia

- Irritability and nervousness
- Menstrual irregularities
- Weight loss

Diet and Thyroid

Your diet can create a sluggish thyroid that will lower your metabolism and cause weight gain. For example, low-fat diets cause high insulin and leptin levels. Leptin has a close relationship with the thyroid. When our ancestors faced starvation, leptin levels would fall, which would tell the thyroid to slow down metabolism. As you eat more sugars and refined carbohydrates, you create insulin resistance and leptin resistance, so even though those levels are high, your body is not listening to them. Therefore, if you're overweight, your thyroid gland might be directed to keep your weight high because it thinks the leptin levels are low.

As you can see, maintaining a healthy thyroid is very important. You can make a great impact on the function of your thyroid by focusing on your toxin exposures, diet, and stress levels, which would improve your metabolism and allow you to lose weight. A diet low in sugars and refined carbohydrates and high in vegetables, lean proteins, and healthy fats will give you the nutrients you need to support your thyroid.

TRUSTY TIP

If you've been diagnosed with Hashimoto's thyroiditis, you might want to consider a six-month trial of a gluten-free diet to see whether you feel better.

Estrogen/Progesterone

Estrogen and progesterone are known as the female hormones. However, men also have these hormones, but in smaller amounts than women do. Estrogen has more than 400 functions in your body, including increasing your metabolic rate and improving your insulin sensitivity. Progesterone is also a very important hormone because it balances estrogen, has a calming effect, builds bone, and slows the digestive process, among other things.

Estrogens are produced throughout the body, especially in the ovaries, adrenals, fat cells, and placenta (in pregnant women). People actually produce three major types of estrogen: estrone (E1), estradiol (E2), and estriol (E3). Each of these molecules has different levels of activity, so when they bind to the estrogen receptors in cells, they produce different levels of effect.

Since estrogen has so many functions in our body, there are many symptoms that occur if the level is too low. Some of the most common symptoms (as you'll see in the following list) are related to the skin, bone density, memory, and weight gain.

Symptoms of low estrogen include:

- Decreased memory

- Increased cholesterol and insulin resistance

- Low libido

- Osteoporosis

- Reduced breast size, acne, oily skin, wrinkles, and vaginal dryness

- Stress incontinence

Progesterone

Progesterone comes from cholesterol and serves as a precursor to the production of other hormones such as cortisol, testosterone, and estrogen. In women prior to menopause, it's produced in the ovaries by the corpus luteum cyst. This cyst occurs every month after a woman ovulates. This is one of the reasons why regular ovulation and hormone cycles are important. If you're not regularly ovulating, you may be getting inadequate amounts of progesterone and not appropriately balancing estrogen (the symptoms of which are in the following list). After menopause, some progesterone is made in your adrenal glands.

Symptoms of low progesterone include:

- Anxiety, irritability, and depression
- Insomnia

- Osteoporosis
- PMS, heavy menses, and/or irregular menses

Progesterone is important because it helps to balance estrogen. Estrogen tends to stimulate growth in cells, especially those of the breast and uterus, and progesterone stabilizes that growth. You need both of these things to happen in your body—growth and stabilization. As you age, progesterone production decreases.

In addition to balancing estrogen, progesterone has a number of other good effects. Among other things, it aids weight loss and helps the body use and eliminate fats, increases the metabolic rate, helps thyroid hormone function, and acts as a natural diuretic to remove extra fluid from the body. As seen in the following lists, even though it has many wonderful functions, too much of a good thing like progesterone can lead to increased insulin resistance and weight gain.

Functions of natural progesterone include:

- Acts as an antidepressant
- Balances estrogen
- Builds bone
- Calms/anti-anxiety
- Diuretic
- Helps thyroid hormone function

- Helps with sleep
- Improves libido
- Increases metabolic rate
- Lowers blood pressure and cholesterol
- Protects against breast cancer

Symptoms of too much progesterone include:

- Bloating
- Increases appetite and carbohydrate cravings

- Increases cortisol, fat storage, and insulin resistance
- Lowers growth hormone

How Estrogen and Progesterone Work

E2 is a type of estrogen that you have in higher quantity when you're young. It increases your metabolic rate, helps with insulin sensitivity, lowers blood pressure, gives you favorable cholesterol ratios, and generally helps keep you lean. It also enhances the production of the hormone serotonin, which helps to regulate hunger.

As women go through menopause and ovarian function decreases, E2 production is reduced and E1 becomes the main source of estrogen. This is a problem because E1 is made from body fat and the adrenals. As E1 takes over, it begins to shift the fat from your hips and buttocks over to your belly. The fat on your buttocks and hips actually helps with insulin sensitivity. When it's shifted over to your belly, you lose some of your curves and gain more belly fat.

This starts a vicious cycle because the more E1 you have, the more belly fat you produce, and that fat ends up making more E1. As a result, you gain weight that becomes very difficult to lose. Another problem with E1 when compared with E2 is that E2 helps with insulin sensitivity, and E1 creates insulin resistance, which puts you behind the eight ball because insulin resistance adds even more belly fat!

It's important to make sure that your estrogen levels are balanced with enough progesterone and testosterone. Because of these vicious cycles, postmenopausal women who are overweight can have 50 to 100 times as much estrogen in their bodies as women of normal weight. These higher levels are often not appropriately balanced with progesterone and can lead to a number of symptoms.

Symptoms of estrogen imbalance (too much estrogen) include:

- Belly fat
- Bloating
- Carb cravings
- Cervical dysplasia
- Decreased sexual interest

- Depression with anxiety, mood swings, and panic attacks
- Dizziness
- Fibrocystic breast and swollen breast, joint stiffness, hair loss, and dry skin

- Headaches
- Heavy periods, uterine fibroids, and hot flashes
- Impaired memory
- Incontinence

- Increased risk of breast cancer, cancer of the uterus, and autoimmune diseases
- Insomnia/fatigue and night sweats
- Weight gain (especially abdomen, hips, and thighs)

The ratio between estrogen and progesterone is important for a number of reasons, including maintaining optimal body weight. The hormones work together to control the way the body releases insulin and stores fat. E2 tends to increase insulin sensitivity and reduce fat storage while progesterone, in general, has the opposite effect.

TRUSTY TIP

If you use over-the-counter progesterone cream, don't use too much of it, or you may contribute to increased fat storage. On the other hand, if you have too much estrogen in relationship to progesterone, your risk for bleeding, breast cysts, breast cancer, and endometrial cancer may increase. With hormones, it's all about balance!

Estrogen and Progesterone in Men

Estrogen and progesterone also play an important part in the metabolism of men. Both men and women have progesterone as a precursor, or building block, for their other steroid hormones, cortisol, testosterone, and estrogen. Men normally make much more testosterone than women. However, when they have an increase in stress or poor diet, as they increase belly fat, they start to increase the conversion of their testosterone to estrogen.

Men need some estrogen; it helps with their libido and protects their hearts. However, they only need a small amount, and the more belly fat they have, the more estrogen they make. Eventually, higher levels of estrogen in men can create problems with erectile dysfunction, decreased libido, reduced sperm count, depression, weight gain, and other problems. Progesterone in men also helps in balancing the estrogen that they have, and it keeps them from turning their testosterone into dihydrotestosterone (DHT). DHT is a stronger form of testosterone and has been associated with prostate enlargement, so you don't want too much. However, since there are no "good" hormones and no "bad" hormones, it's helpful to have some DHT around to enhance libido for men.

Testosterone

Testosterone is commonly known as "the male hormone." Although it's present in large amounts in men and is responsible for most of the masculine qualities, it's necessary for women as well. Testosterone is needed to maintain muscle mass and strength, bone mass, overall sense of well-being, libido, and, in men, sperm production. Since the amount of muscle you have is directly related to your metabolism, having enough testosterone to build muscle mass will increase your metabolism and help you to lose weight.

In men, testosterone is produced mainly in the testes, but also in the adrenals. In women, testosterone comes mainly from the adrenals but also from the ovaries.

Testosterone and Men

Testosterone is an anabolic or building-up hormone, and the highest levels in men are found after puberty and when they're in their 20s. A natural decline in testosterone levels occurs each decade after the 20s. As a matter of fact, half of healthy men between the ages of 50 and 70 have testosterone levels below the lowest level seen in healthy men 20 to 40 years of age.

Over the past few decades, the rate of testosterone decline has accelerated. In 2006, Dr. Travison in the *Journal of Clinical Endocrinology Metabolism* showed that there is a population level decline in testosterone for every age group in men, which can't be explained by a natural decline in testosterone alone. This means that for all men in a certain age group (20s, 30s, 40s, etc.), the average level of testosterone for all the men is lower than it would have been for men in that same age group 40 or 50 years ago. Why is this happening? Testosterone levels are closely related to diet, stress and cortisol levels, lifestyle, and toxin exposure.

Because testosterone production is related to many aspects of a man's (or woman's) life, many things can cause a reduction in production. Many diseases and nutrient depletions lower testosterone production.

Things that lower testosterone production include:

- Aging
- Anabolic steroids
- Diabetes
- Excess alcohol
- Excess estrogen
- High refined carbohydrate diet
- Insulin resistance
- Low progesterone

- Obesity/body fat
- Ovarian removal/surgery in women and testicular trauma/surgery in men
- Pituitary tumor (prolactinoma)
- Sedentary lifestyle
- Sleep disturbances
- Statin medications (if cholesterol reduced too far)
- Stress
- Tobacco use and toxin exposure
- Zinc deficiency

As you eat more refined carbohydrates, sugars, and high fructose corn syrup, you create an imbalance in insulin and cortisol, which leads to decreased testosterone production. This combination increases belly fat, and because belly fat has the aromatase enzyme to turn testosterone into estrogen, the amount of testosterone is reduced even further. A vicious cycle takes place when there is more belly fat and weight gain, more inflammation and cortisol demand, less testosterone production, and less muscle mass development followed by lower metabolism, leading to increased belly fat. Besides the symptoms of low testosterone, signs of excess estrogen in men include enlarged breasts and increased fat deposits in the hips and thighs.

We talked about many of the diseases, stressors, and nutrient depletions that could lead to reduced testosterone production. However, many men have symptoms of reduced testosterone that are actually a result of elevated estrogens blocking the effects of testosterone. Belly fat definitely causes an increase in estrogen in men and women. But many people don't realize that their medications can have the same effect. If you take any of these medications regularly, take the quiz in Chapter 15 to see if you have any further symptoms of low testosterone or estrogen excess.

Medications or drugs that can increase estrogen in men include:

- Alcohol, amphetamines, cocaine, and marijuana
- Antacids
- Anti-inflammatory medications, antidepressants, antifungal medications, antipsychotic medications, and blood pressure medications
- Antibiotics (sulfa medications, penicillins, erythromycins, toxins, isoniazid)

Low testosterone has many symptoms. The most common are fatigue, irritability, weight gain, loss of muscle mass despite working out, low libido, increased cholesterol, sleep disturbance, and erectile dysfunction.

When men go to their physicians with any of these symptoms, they are often given separate medications to treat the symptoms rather than an evaluation and treatment for low testosterone.

Testosterone supplementation is being used to help many men. However, it requires close supervision of a physician trained in this type of medicine. It is imperative to have initial laboratory testing done to diagnose a deficiency, use only bioidentical testosterone, replace the testosterone only to your normal levels, and continue following laboratory levels closely to monitor the effects of testosterone. In addition, testosterone replacement needs to be accompanied by the appropriate diet, stress management, lifestyle changes, and reduction in toxin exposure.

Many men often confuse the symptoms of low testosterone with "old age." However, since chronically low testosterone is associated with diseases like diabetes, metabolic syndrome, depression, osteoporosis, and heart disease, if you have many of the following symptoms, speak to your physician and ask to have your testosterone levels checked.

Symptoms of low testosterone include:

- Anxiety, irritability, and depression
- Belly fat
- Erectile dysfunction, low libido, and decreased intensity of orgasm
- Fatigue
- High blood sugar and/or high cholesterol
- Loss of memory
- Low muscle mass
- Osteoporosis
- Weight gain

Testosterone and Women

Women need testosterone to build their lean muscle mass and bone mass. The same factors that reduce testosterone in men can contribute to low testosterone in women. Women with low testosterone may be fatigued, have low bone mass or muscle mass, and have a low libido. Another important thing for women to consider is that women with low testosterone might be at an increased risk for breast cancer. Evidence shows that testosterone also helps balance estrogen in women. On the other hand, syndromes such as polycystic ovarian syndrome (PCOS) create a situation in which too much testosterone is produced. These women tend to have acne, excess hair growth on their faces, irregular menses, infertility, and weight gain. A connection exists between polycystic ovarian syndrome and insulin resistance as well. The best way to manage testosterone levels is to maintain a diet such as the hormone weight-loss diet, which reduces insulin demand.

DHEA

DHEA is a hormone made mostly by your adrenal glands, with a small amount being produced by your brain and your skin. It's one of the most plentiful hormones in the body, and it's an anabolic, or building-up, hormone. However, DHEA is another one of the hormones that starts declining in your 20s; by the age of 70, you make about one fourth the amount you made early in your life. DHEA is made from the building block hormone pregnenolone (which is derived from cholesterol) and is a precursor to estrogen and testosterone.

Originally, it was thought that DHEA was just a building block for estrogen and testosterone. However, special receptors for DHEA were found on cells in the liver, kidneys, and testes so it was determined to have its own functions as well. DHEA has some functions that are related to weight loss. It naturally increases the hormone serotonin, which helps with satiety and enhances insulin sensitivity. Animal studies have shown that DHEA can help in the prevention of obesity. DHEA production is very sensitive to stress and is one of the first hormones to be depleted during times of high cortisol demand.

DHEA is more than just a precursor to estrogen and testosterone. It has uses throughout the body that are detailed in the following list.

DHEA functions include:

- Bone growth
- Brain function/improve memory
- Decreases cholesterol
- Immune support

- Increases sense of well-being
- Insulin sensitivity
- Muscle maintenance
- Stress response
- Tissue repair and maintenance

DHEA is available as an over-the-counter supplement. However, it's important to know your hormone status before taking DHEA or any other hormones. I strongly recommend testing to determine what your various hormone levels are. If you take DHEA and have adrenal fatigue or low cortisol, DHEA supplementation can further reduce your cortisol production and make you feel worse. Also, make sure that what you're taking is a high-quality DHEA. I recommend pharmaceutical-grade supplements that are available through practitioners. (See Appendix C for further information.)

Symptoms of low DHEA include:

- Anxiety and depression
- Sleep disturbance and fatigue
- Insulin resistance
- Joint aches
- Low libido
- Low sense of well-being
- Obesity
- Poor immune response
- Poor stress response

Symptoms of too much DHEA include:

- Anger, irritability, mood changes, and depression
- Acne, deepening of voice, facial hair, and oily skin
- Fatigue/insomnia
- Sugar cravings
- Weight gain

One of the best ways to maintain an optimal level of DHEA is to reduce your cortisol demand. This means eating in a way that will reduce insulin demand and subsequent cortisol demand, managing stress, getting adequate sleep, and eliminating toxins. The less your body has to shift the building blocks from making DHEA to making cortisol, the more hormone you will have available to take care of tissue growth and repair and the production of the other anabolic hormones, testosterone and estrogen. The seven principles of the diet in Part 2 are an excellent way to accomplish that goal.

Human Growth Hormone

Human growth hormone (HGH) is very important for overall balance in your body. It's produced in a small gland in the brain called the pituitary gland. HGH has many wonderful properties including building muscle and bone, burning fat, increasing immunity, and improving your health in general. The body's production of HGH starts to decline naturally after your 20s. This is why, as you get older, you may start to accumulate fat even if you haven't changed your diet or physical activity.

Growth hormone improves your metabolism by increasing your muscle mass. It helps your body absorb amino acids, the building blocks for protein and muscle; helps build muscle; and prevents muscle breakdown. It's also instrumental in reducing your fat stores. HGH also encourages fat cells to break down. And it reduces fat storage by communicating with fat cells and by reducing insulin's ability to put sugar into them.

Symptoms of low growth hormone include:

- Decreased muscle mass and muscle strength
- Depression
- Low libido
- High insulin
- Insomnia/sleep disturbance/fatigue
- Short stature
- Wrinkles

In addition to the fact that growth hormone naturally decreases in production after their 20s, people often accelerate that reduction by eating a diet with refined carbohydrates that increases insulin and body fat, both of which suppress the production of growth hormone. In other words, the more body fat a person has, the less HGH he has.

Another way you can significantly reduce production is from sleep deprivation. Growth hormone is released in adults in pulses about five times a day. The highest production of growth hormone is within the first 90 minutes of the sleep cycle. If you have difficulty falling asleep or staying asleep, you may further reduce its production.

Things that reduce growth hormone production include:

- Alcohol
- Excess dietary fat
- Excess estrogen
- Excess insulin
- High blood sugar
- High cortisol
- Sedentary lifestyle
- Sleep disturbance
- Stress
- Toxins

The Least You Need to Know

- There are no "good" hormones or "bad" hormones. They each have their own functions and work best when appropriately balanced.
- Estrogen works to enhance metabolism and reduce insulin resistance. But too much estrogen, as seen in obesity, can increase the risk of some cancers.

- Testosterone has many important functions. Low testosterone is associated with cardiovascular disease, diabetes, erectile dysfunction, osteoporosis, and depression in men.

- If you have symptoms of hormone imbalance, have your hormone levels tested by a reputable physician.

- If you're considering taking hormone replacements, make sure to take bioidentical hormones.

Losing Weight with Healthy Hormones

Toxins can create hormone imbalance and weight gain. Instead of being overwhelmed by these toxins, it's important to understand exactly where you find them and how you can avoid them. This part starts with a chapter about how to reduce your exposure to toxins to help you lose weight, balance your hormones, and improve your overall health. You'll also learn about the different kinds of nutrients we have to take in every day and how to make the best use of them.

Many of us don't appreciate the effect that our hormone balance has on our weight and our ability to lose it. Unbalanced hormones can make you fat. This part explains bioidentical hormones and how they relate to men and women.

One of the central issues regarding the obesity epidemic, aside from improper diet, is a number of different stressors we are faced with every day, so in this part of the book, you look at the impact of stress on your weight. And we all know that exercise is important for weight loss and overall health. This part also looks at how you can build muscle and reverse metabolic decline.

Finally, this part looks at the fact that we are social beings who rely on each other for support and feedback.

Principle #1: Eliminate Toxins

In This Chapter

- What toxins are
- What toxins do to your hormones
- How toxins make you gain weight
- Specific toxins explored

As you'll see in this chapter, Tom's experience as a farmer is a great example of the importance of eliminating toxins from what we eat and what we breathe. But many are not aware that toxins can cause weight gain. In fact, toxins can play such an important role in weight gain that I have made it the number one principle in the hormone weight-loss diet. This chapter explains why.

Tom's Story

Tom came to see me a number of years ago. He is a jovial, 53-year-old man who has worked on his family's farm for 40 years. He has owned it for the last 20 years. Tom's farm is a large producer of corn and cattle, and he worked in almost every capacity there over four decades. Ten years ago, when the economy tanked, Tom worked even longer hours than usual trying to make ends meet and to improve productivity. He ate many meals on the run from fast-food restaurants in Styrofoam containers, and would often eat only candy bars during the day while he was in the fields.

Over the next five years, Tom worked to improve the situation on the farm in spite of the economy. He became increasingly fatigued and gained 10 pounds.

Tom became interested in organic farming and a more holistic lifestyle. He began focusing on stress reduction and changing his farm over to an organic farm. He took up a hobby of making stained glass and felt much more relaxed as he was working in his shop. Overall, he felt like he was living a better lifestyle.

However, over the past year, Tom has been even more tired. He has also noticed lower muscle mass, has had difficulty sleeping, has gained 30 pounds, has been feeling muscle aches, and has had a lower libido. This was the point at which he came to see me.

First, I took a detailed history of Tom's health problems, diet, work history, and lifestyle. One of the things that stuck out was his occupation as a farmer and long history of exposure to pesticides for 35 years. In addition, as his stress levels increased and he was eating more poor-quality food, he was exposed to the toxins in Styrofoam and was consuming a lot of trans fats and high fructose corn syrup.

Tom's most significant symptoms came after he started working with stained glass, which exposed him to lead. The addition of lead to his list of offenders was too much for his body to detoxify.

The results of Tom's blood tests showed that his liver was stressed, and his lead level was high. I referred him to a specialist for removal of the lead, and Tom removed all lead from his house. I also prescribed maintaining a whole food diet and getting as much gentle exercise as he could manage. I added adequate sleep and nutrients to support his liver, which is responsible for removing lead from the body. (See Chapter 12 for a list of those nutrients.)

After six months on this routine, Tom's lead level was significantly reduced, his cholesterol and blood sugar were normal, and he had lost 25 pounds. I explained to him that all of the toxins he was exposed to were additive, and that his liver had become so overwhelmed, it was unable to remove them adequately. Now, he works very hard to avoid toxin exposure, including limiting his use of products containing phthalates. Tom continues to take care of himself, his weight has returned to normal, he has regained his energy, and the rest of his symptoms have gone away.

What Are Toxins?

Toxins are poisons that can affect your body internally or externally. They can be chemicals that occur naturally or in a synthetic form. More than 120,000 man-made chemicals have been brought into the environment, and this number grows each year. Most of them have never been tested for safety.

DEFINITION

A **toxin** is a poisonous substance produced by living cells or organisms.

Toxins confuse our metabolisms. Additives and processed foods, such as refined sugar and high fructose corn syrup, create strain on our livers and detoxification systems because our bodies try to handle foods (or body fill) they were not designed to use. In addition, many of these additives—such as hydrogenated fats, high fructose corn syrup, artificial sweeteners, flavor enhancers, and preservatives—do not contain nutrients. The result is we are eating foods that add calories without providing nutrition and, on top of that, we are creating a hormone imbalance. And I haven't yet mentioned the pesticides in our food!

In your everyday life, the majority of toxins you're exposed to are not by your choice. You breathe them in, unknowingly drink them with your colas, absorb them through your feet when you walk on the carpets in your home, and much more.

DID YOU KNOW?

A report released by the Centers for Disease Control in 2009 found detectable levels of a total of 212 chemicals in blood or urine samples of 2,400 people nationwide. Little is known about the effects of most of these chemicals on humans.

Environmental Toxins

In the last hundred years, people have been exposed to an unprecedented load of toxins, including pesticides, industrial chemicals, heavy metals, and more. These toxins have accumulated and exceeded the average body's ability to get rid of them. Studies have shown that many common toxins promote obesity.

New research suggests that being exposed to numerous toxins may be more dangerous than originally thought. However, the good news is that your body also is very good at getting rid of them. In addition, if you can learn to recognize where toxins are and how to avoid them, you can reduce your overall exposure to them.

Bisphenol A

Bisphenol A (BPA) is a known environmental estrogen. It's used to make polycarbonate plastics and the resin that is used for most food and beverage cans, dental sealants, baby bottles, water bottles, and many other products. It's one of the highest-volume chemicals produced worldwide.

In 2003, more than 6.4 billion pounds of BPA was produced, with a 6 to 10 percent growth in demand expected per year! Heat and contact with either acidic or basic compounds release the BPA in containers into food.

A large amount of BPA leaches from landfills into the surrounding ecosystem. One study showed that 95 percent of urine samples from people in the United States examined by the Centers for Disease Control had measurable BPA levels. This is consistent with the findings from other countries. BPA is rapidly metabolized, so these findings suggest that human exposure to significant amounts of BPA must be continuous and from multiple sources.

A study done with students at Harvard University looked at the level of BPA in the urine of students as compared to how much they drank out of plastic water bottles. The students were given either stainless-steel bottles or polycarbonate bottles to drink clear liquids for four weeks at a time. Urine samples taken at the beginning of the study compared to samples taken after a week using the stainless-steel bottles showed a significant reduction in BPA. The students then were instructed to start drinking out of the polycarbonate bottles again, and the levels of BPA in their urine increased to the same level as when the study started.

These results show that you can make an impact on the amount of toxins you have in your body. This is important because in 2007, a group of 38 experts on BPA concluded that the average levels of BPA that people have in their bodies is above those that that could cause harm to animals in laboratory experiments. Because of these results, some bicarbonate bottle manufacturers voluntarily eliminated BPA from their products. In 2008, Canada imposed a ban on the use of BPA in polycarbonate baby bottles. Similar legislation is being considered in several U.S. states.

Phthalates

Phthalates are used as plasticizers and are found in personal care items such as makeup, shampoo, moisturizer, hairspray, and cologne. They are also found in detergents, cleaning materials, modeling clay, paints, children's toys, and food packaging. When you smell a vinyl shower curtain or notice that new car scent, those are phthalates leaching from the plastic into the air.

Phthalates are currently being studied as an anti-androgen, which means they work against hormones like testosterone. Several of these compounds have caused reduced sperm count and other signs of low testosterone. (Low testosterone is connected to weight gain and decreased muscle mass in women and men.) Some studies have also linked phthalates to liver cancer.

The Environmental Working Group has focused on phthalates since 1998 and, in 2003, they published the Body Burden Study. They found 210 industrial and consumer product chemicals—among them a half dozen phthalates—in nine Americans who agreed to submit their blood and urine for analysis. In July 2008, as a result of pressure from the Environmental Working Group and other health groups, the U.S. Congress passed legislation banning six phthalates from cosmetics and children's toys.

DID YOU KNOW?

Because people are exposed to so many them, at any given time 84 percent of the U.S. population is contaminated with at least six different phthalates!

There are many different kinds of phthalates. According to FreeDrinkingwater.com, the exact amount of phthalates produced each year varies from source to source. According to one estimate, the phthalates volume manufactured worldwide in 1999 was about 10 billion pounds (valued at $5 billion), with an average annual growth rate of 2 to 3 percent.

Experts believe that the actions of phthalates are cumulative. Over the past eight years, a series of scientific studies showed that the U.S. population has a chronic exposure to numerous phthalates. The studies linked the chemicals to birth defects in boys, reproductive problems in men, and thyroid problems in both men and women.

Low thyroid means lower metabolism and an increased chance for weight gain. Also, the immune system is affected by phthalates, which can be associated with illnesses such as allergies, asthma, and contact dermatitis. Anytime an increase occurs in inflammation or cortisol demand, there is a corresponding increased risk of belly fat, weight gain, and severe hormone imbalance. It's going to be more and more important for people to monitor and reduce the amount of phthalates in the environment.

Toxins in Our Food

The toxins in our food come from many sources: pesticides, antibiotics, artificial sweeteners, high fructose corn syrup, and trans fats, to name a few. Many times, the food you eat to provide nutrients for your body contains toxins that put stress on your liver, kidneys, and other organs in your body. The more you learn about them, the more you will be able to limit your exposure to them.

Pesticides

The pesticides that are sprayed on crops end up in your food and drinks and therefore in your body with potentially harmful effects. And many researchers believe that the pesticides in your food place you at higher risk for insulin resistance, metabolic syndrome, diabetes, and obesity.

Consider these research findings:

- The Environmental Protection Agency began monitoring human exposure to toxic environmental chemicals in 1970. Five of what are noted as the most toxic chemicals humans have ever created were found in 100 percent of all samples. Nine more chemicals were found in 91 to 98 percent of the samples.

- Another study based in Michigan found *DDT* in more than 70 percent of 4-year-olds. This fact is curious because DDT has been banned since 1972!

DEFINITION

DDT (dichlorodiphenyltrichloroethane) is a well-known synthetic pesticide that was widely used from 1950 to 1980. It has been found to be related to diabetes, cancer, genetic damage, and endocrine disruption. In 1972, DDT was banned in the United States. As of 2007, India is the only country that still allows the use of DDT.

- A study done by the National Institutes of Health looked at 30,000 farm workers who use pesticides. The research shows that if the workers used one of seven specific pesticides, they had a significantly increased risk of diabetes.

- A study published in *Diabetes Care* looked at 2,016 people and found that 80 percent had detectable levels of six common persistent organic pollutants (POP). They found higher concentrations in older people and in women. Of the various groups compared, people with the highest levels of POP were 38 times more likely to have diabetes than people with the lowest levels.

Just because a pesticide was banned doesn't mean that you can't be exposed to it. In many areas in this country, the soil is still contaminated with residues of the pesticides we banned years ago. In addition, many of the fruits for sale in large supermarkets come from countries that don't have the same restrictions on pesticides as the United States. Because many toxic chemicals are stored in fat tissue, many animal products can be concentrated sources of pesticides and toxins.

DID YOU KNOW?

The Environmental Working Group identified 12 plants with the highest level of pesticides. These are peaches, celery, apples, nectarines, sweet bell peppers, strawberries, cherries, pears, lettuce, spinach, grapes, and potatoes. It's therefore important to buy these from organic suppliers if possible.

Artificial Sweeteners and High Fructose Corn Syrup

Any food that has an "artificial" label should not go into your body. The food many eat is chemically altered to promote shelf life and increase consumption, not nurture the body. For example, the artificial sweeteners used in food are actually worse than sugar. These sweeteners are man-made chemicals and are not recognized as food.

Aspartame (Equal) breaks down into methyl alcohol, a chemical that is poisonous to the human body. It's associated with a number of side effects, including decreased vision, hearing impairment, seizures, migraines, memory loss, irritability, anxiety, hives, and hyperactivity. Sucralose (Splenda) has been linked to migraines and low thyroid.

High fructose corn syrup is one of the worst toxic offenders. It's almost identical to table sugar! In fact, I think of it as a "supersugar." It's found in almost everything these days, including soft drinks. Before the 1970s, it wasn't even in the food supply.

The syrup causes changes in the liver by increasing the amount of glucose or sugar it absorbs, which makes the liver hungry for more sugar. This process accelerates insulin resistance and obesity, and it leads to resistance of the hormone leptin, which helps control the appetite. Therefore, you're more likely to have insulin resistance and become obese, but remain hungry. Sadly, Tufts University reports that Americans consume more calories from high fructose corn syrup than from any other source.

Hydrogenated Oils

Hydrogenated oils, also called trans fats, come from soy, so you might think they are good for you. Not! They are manufactured in laboratories into toxic foods that are not recognized by the human body.

Trans fats are dangerous to your metabolism because they bind to receptors on your cells that slow fat burning. They also increase cholesterol levels and the risk of insulin resistance.

Hydrogenated oils have absolutely no nutritional value. Part of their popularity stems from the fact that they are inert, so they don't turn rancid like butter or vegetable oil. This increases their shelf lives, but when you consume them, they cause damage to your metabolism, leading to weight gain.

Trans fats are used as a preservative in almost every food on grocery store shelves, so it's important to shop in the perimeter where the "whole" foods are.

TRUSTY TIP

Look for the words "partially hydrogenated oil" or "shortening" on ingredient lists to tell whether a food has trans fats in it. Also, look on the nutrition labels to see if they list any trans fats.

One interesting thing about food labels is that food companies are allowed to state "zero trans fats" if they have under 0.5 gram of trans fat per serving. This may not sound like a big deal. However, if you eat a few servings a day, you could be taking in 2 or 3 grams of trans fat per day. Again, you might say "big deal!" But it really is. An analysis of several studies in 2006 by Dr. Mozaffarian showed that increasing your intake of trans fats by 2 percent increased your risk of heart disease by 23 percent! Therefore, even if the package says "zero trans fats," if you see "partially hydrogenated oils" on the ingredients list, it has some trans fats.

Refined Sugars and Carbohydrates

Refined carbohydrates and sugars are everywhere—white bread, sugar, pasta, white rice, and white potatoes. These foods are all quickly absorbed into the bloodstream, which causes a rapid increase in blood sugar and a high demand for insulin.

Grains are refined to help extend their shelf lives. In the refining process, the bran and the germ of the grain are removed, which means that its fiber, vitamins, and minerals are also removed. The result is a "food" with minimal nutritional value, which causes a rapid rise in blood sugar.

Other Toxins

Three other potential toxins to be aware of are caffeine, some drugs, and tobacco.

Caffeine is found in products such as coffee, tea, soda, and chocolate. Caffeine acts as a central nervous system stimulant and is actually the world's most widely consumed psychoactive substance. However, unlike many other psychoactive substances, it's legal and unregulated in nearly all areas.

All stimulants can cause insulin resistance and adrenal stress, which can contribute to weight gain. If caffeine is used in large amounts over an extended period of time, it can lead to a condition known as caffeinism, which combines caffeine dependency with a number of other symptoms such as nervousness, anxiety, insomnia, and headaches. Even lower doses of caffeine can contribute to sleep disturbance, which contributes to weight gain.

Some studies, such as the one published in *Obesity Research* in 2005, demonstrate increased weight loss due to increased *thermogenesis* with high caffeine consumption. However, a study done in 2011 in the *Journal of Nutrition* shows that caffeine reduces glucose tolerance in men. Therefore, the risk of insulin resistance is increased. Another study from 2011 seen in the *Journal of Nutrition* showed that caffeine consumption prevented cortisol in the blood from returning to its normal levels in healthy men. Any potential increase in weight loss by expending more energy might eventually be reduced due to glucose intolerance and cortisol elevation.

 DEFINITION

Thermogenesis is the process of heat production in warm-blooded animals. It requires energy and increases the expenditure of calories.

Illicit drugs are certainly thought of as toxins. However, some prescription drugs can create weight gain as well. Drugs affect us all differently, so it's important to see how you react to the medications you take and whether they cause you to gain weight. Never stop taking any drug without consulting with your doctor first!

No one knows for sure why, but prescription drugs used to treat mood disorders, seizures, migraines, diabetes, and even high blood pressure can cause weight gain. Dr. George Blackburn of Harvard University compiled a list of more than 50 medications with this effect. Some of the most common drugs are prednisone, Elavil, Tofranil, Zyprexa, Paxil, Zoloft, Depakote, DiaBeta, Cardura, Nexium, and Prevacid.

Nonprescription medications can also cause weight gain. Diphenhydramine is found in cold and allergy remedies and sleep aids and is known to increase weight. The fact that these drugs can be associated with weight gain does not mean that they should never be used. However, if you're on one of these prescription or nonprescription medications and have a significant problem with weight gain, speak to your physician about the possibility of changing your medication to one that does not have this association.

Alcohol is another drug that needs to be considered. Although the antioxidant and health benefits of red wine have been demonstrated, drinking red wine still exposes you to a large amount of sugar. In addition, the alcohol must be detoxified in your liver, which puts added stress on it. Phase I of the diet (discussed in Chapter 20) does not allow alcohol.

Tobacco contains many toxins that stress the liver and reduce the body's ability to remove other toxins. For example, the hydrocarbons in tobacco damage cells, and nicotine causes insulin resistance. In addition to developing lung cancer, smokers also have an increased risk of developing type 2 diabetes, osteoporosis, emphysema, and heart disease. If you smoke, do you need any more reasons to quit?

What Toxins Do to Your Hormones

In Chapter 2, I covered the fact that your hormones are the chemical messengers in your body and that your metabolism depends on good hormone balance. Toxins can destroy that balance.

Toxins often act as endocrine disruptors in your body. Endocrine disrupters are any substance that changes the way hormones usually work. They may increase, decrease, or change the activity of the hormone by mimicking it, blocking it, changing the amount of hormone that is produced, or changing the speed at which the hormone works. The hormones that are often affected include estrogen, thyroid hormone, testosterone, cortisol, and insulin. Because they all work together in concert, a problem with any one of these hormones can have far-reaching effects.

For example, you can be exposed to many scents in air fresheners, candles, detergents, or beauty products that have phthalates in their ingredients. Because these toxins are known to reduce the level of testosterone, as a male you can see a reduced sperm count, and as a female you can see a reduction in lean muscle mass that can contribute to weight gain.

Other toxins such as BPA, which is known to increase estrogen, can aggravate problems such as polycystic ovarian syndrome. A study in the *Journal of the American Medical Association* found that those with higher BPA levels in their urine had a 300 percent greater risk of cardiovascular disease and a 240 percent greater risk of diabetes.

Toxins increase weight through different mechanisms. First, it's easy to see how hormone disruptors can wreak havoc on your metabolism. We already know that increases in BPA cause an increase in estrogen. However, it can also cause an increase in insulin levels. As a matter of fact, in as little as four days of exposure to BPA, your pancreas is stimulated to make more insulin. More insulin in your body can lead to insulin resistance, where your body no longer listens to insulin and won't be able to utilize your blood sugar the right way. As you become more insulin resistant, you start to store any sugar that you take in as fat.

BPA has also been shown to directly create obesity. In addition, as different toxins create damage within the body, there is an increase in inflammation that causes an increase in the demand for cortisol, the stress hormone. High levels of cortisol can also cause the body to add fat, which creates weight gain. And high levels of toxins (such as heavy metals) block the signals in your brain for leptin, a hormone that helps control your appetite and tells your brain you're full. If your brain becomes resistant to the effects of leptin, you feel hungry all the time.

Many people with high levels of toxins in their body are obese. One study showed a relationship between blood levels of BPA and body fat in women. This occurs because toxins are stored in the fat cells. And as you accumulate more and more toxins in your body, more and more storage space is needed, and your body holds on to the fat cells. This storage system is a way your body keeps the toxins from circulating. Keep this in mind as you're losing weight, because as you lose fat, you may release some of these toxins. Therefore, you will want to make sure that you're drinking plenty of water to flush your kidneys.

A study in *Obesity Reviews* in 2003 showed that pesticides and polychlorinated biphe-nyls (PCBs) are released from fat tissue when you lose weight and can poison your metabolism, preventing further weight loss. Therefore, it's important for you to keep your liver and kidneys healthy as you lose weight so you can remove these toxins and continue the weight loss. In Chapter 12, I discuss different methods of detoxification that you can use as well as supplements to support your liver and help you detoxify any chemicals released from your fat cells as you lose weight.

The Least You Need to Know

- Toxins often act as endocrine disruptors in the body.
- Pesticides in your food place you at higher risk for insulin resistance, metabolic syndrome, diabetes, and obesity.
- High fructose corn syrup accelerates the process of insulin resistance and obesity, and it leads to resistance of the hormone leptin, which helps control appetite.

- Trans fats are dangerous to your metabolism because, among other things, they bind to receptors on cells that slow fat burning.
- Many people with high levels of toxins in their bodies are obese.

Principle #2: Eat Right

In This Chapter

- How eating some fat can be a good thing
- Determining your essential nutrients
- Using the glycemic index to balance your hormones
- How glycemic load is related to weight control

This chapter describes the basics of healthy nutrition, which you should know in order to keep your hormones balanced. We take a closer look at the importance of the second principle: eat right.

Amy's Story

Amy was 46 years old when we first met. She was at the end of her rope. She worked very hard to maintain her weight, and it seemed like the harder she tried, the more weight she gained. Amy has always been a high achiever and a "rule follower." She graduated from dental school at the top of her class.

Amy didn't believe in fad diets, so she followed the U.S. government's Food Pyramid guidelines. In addition, she counted her calories to make sure that she was in the right range for women with a moderate activity level who want to lose weight. She also ate mainly low-fat or no-fat foods.

Amy went to the gym and walked on the treadmill three to four times a week; she got eight hours of sleep at night; and she did not eat sweets, junk food, or red meat. However, in spite of all the good things she was doing, she was always hungry and her weight kept creeping up. When she went to see her doctor, he noted that her cholesterol was elevated and told her to go on a low-cholesterol diet. She really didn't know how she could possibly take any more fat out of her diet.

When Amy came to see me, she was extremely frustrated. Nothing seemed to be working. When we looked at her diet, we could see that she was eating mainly sugars and refined carbohydrates: bread, pasta, pretzels, and bagels with trans fats and high fructose corn syrup and very little protein or healthy fats. I explained to her how this diet was contributing to insulin resistance and how she was storing all the sugar she was taking in as fat. On top of that, she was creating inflammation, fatigue, and hunger because of the hormone imbalance.

My prescription for Amy was to focus on whole foods like meats; fish; beans; vegetables; a few high-fiber fruits; and healthy fats like nuts, avocados, wild salmon, and olive oil. It took a lot of convincing to get her to eat fats, but she was willing to do anything at that point. In addition, I told her to make sure she didn't have any trans fats or high fructose corn syrup in her diet. Over the course of the next three months, her hunger was reduced, her cravings stopped, her fatigue improved, and she lost 15 pounds. She continues to feel better and better "without any effort."

There is truth to the concept "you are what you eat." Like a builder who uses substandard materials for construction, a body that is built with poor nutrition might look okay for a while on the outside but will be unable to weather major storms because of how the inside is constructed. And, as in Amy's case, if nutrition continues to be poor, even the outside of the body shows wear and tear. Eventually, chronic disease sets in.

How the Food Pyramids Fooled Us

In 1960, the American Heart Association published the first official endorsement of low-fat, low-cholesterol diet as a means to prevent heart disease. A debate ensued over the next 30 years among physicians and scientists about the ability of the heart-healthy diet to actually prevent heart disease. Despite an overwhelming lack of evidence, the low-fat, low-cholesterol diet became the dogma for good health.

In 1992, the United States produced the first Food Guide Pyramid, which focused on four food groups: breads and cereals, fruits and vegetables, dairy products, meats and fish, and fats and oils.

Dr. Diane Schwarzbein, in her book *The Schwarzbein Principle*, states that the main problem with the limited fats in the pyramid is that unsaturated fats from natural sources can actually aid in weight loss, reduce heart disease, lower blood sugar, and even lower cholesterol. Fats help keep the blood sugar stable and enhance brain function. The government recently updated and released the Food Guide Pyramid based on new data. The main focus of the pyramid remains on grain and dairy products with fruits and vegetables coming next. Meats, nuts, and beans have a small fraction of the pyramid, and fats and oils have a tiny sliver.

DID YOU KNOW?

The concept of a "heart healthy diet" was born in the 1950s. In his book *Good Calories, Bad Calories,* Gary Taubes notes that the country had become fascinated with heart disease in 1955, when President Eisenhower had a heart attack. Interestingly, the president's cholesterol level was 165 (a desirable level) when he had his first heart attack. After following a low-cholesterol, low-fat diet for five years, his cholesterol level was 259 (a high-risk level).

It's interesting that as our country has followed this diet, we have had an alarming increase in the rate of obesity, insulin resistance, and diabetes. As a nation, we have more disease due to chronic inflammation than we have ever seen. In *The Paleo Solution,* Robb Wolf states that the single most important event in all human history is the agricultural revolution. If you look at human history on a relative scale that is 100 yards long, walking 99.5 yards would represent all human history except for the last 5,000 years or so. The last 10,000 years was the time when we transitioned from hunting and gathering to agriculture.

Because our genetics are nearly identical to those of our early ancestors from 100,000 to 200,000 years ago, we are genetically wired to have a nutrient-dense, protein-rich diet that is varied and changes with location and season. Now, we have a diet that is dependent on a few starchy crops such as wheat and corn. These crops can provide a fraction of the vitamins and minerals found in fruits, vegetables, and lean meats.

Many people cannot tolerate the *gluten* found in wheat, rye, and barley. People with a genetic intolerance are noted as having celiac disease and become very ill when they're exposed to gluten. However, many more are just sensitive to gluten and, when they eat it, they develop irritation in their intestines which then creates inflammation, increased cortisol demand, and the possibility of inflammation and autoimmune disease. The gluten reaction can create hormone imbalance. As you will see, my hormone weight-loss diet is different from the "average" diet. For the first 30 days, you will have no grains, and you will focus on lean meats, vegetables, some high-fiber fruits, nuts, and beans. After the first 30 days, you can try adding back some gluten-free whole grains such as quinoa and brown rice.

DEFINITION

Gluten (from the Latin word for glue) is a storage protein that appears in foods processed from wheat and related species, including barley and rye.

Essential Nutrients

Nutrients that the body cannot manufacture in sufficient amounts but are necessary for survival are known as essential nutrients. All humans require the same set of essential nutrients, but the amount needed varies by age, body size, gender, genetic traits, growth, illness, lifestyle habits, and medication use. The essential nutrients we need are as follows:

- Carbohydrates
- Some amino acids (histidine, isoleucine, leucine, lysine, methionine, phenyl alanine, threonine, tryptophan, and valine)
- Essential fatty acids (linoleic acid and alpha-linolenic acid)
- Vitamins
- Minerals
- Water

DEFINITION

Nutrients are chemical substances in food that the body uses to support growth, tissue maintenance and repair, and ongoing health.

Vitamins

Vitamins are chemicals in foods that perform specific functions in the body. Thirteen vitamins have been discovered to this date. They are as follows:

- Vitamin A
- Vitamin C
- Vitamin D
- Vitamin E
- Vitamin K

- B vitamins
  - Thiamine
  - Riboflavin
  - Niacin
  - Pantothenic acid
  - Biotin
  - Vitamin B_6
  - Vitamin B_{12}
  - Folate

Vitamins are either fat-soluble or water-soluble. The B-complex vitamins and vitamin C are soluble in water and are found dissolved in the water in foods. Vitamins A, E, D, and K are considered to be fat-soluble vitamins and are present in the fat portions of food. Except for vitamin B_{12}, water-soluble vitamin stores in the body are limited. If you do not consume enough of them, your body will be deficient within a few weeks to a few months.

Fat-soluble vitamins are stored in the fat tissue of the body and in the liver. These stores are less likely to run out quickly if you stop consuming them. However, one of the dangers with extreme low-fat diets, weight-loss surgery, and fat-blocking medication is that the dieter might have significantly reduced intake or absorption of the fat-soluble vitamins. This can create long-term depletion and health problems due to vitamin deficiency.

Vitamins do not provide energy or serve as structural components of the body. Some play roles as co-enzymes (substances that help enzymes function in your body) in the chemical changes of metabolism. Therefore, if you don't have the appropriate vitamins, your body will not be able to burn fat and sugars for energy the way it needs to, and you will not be able to lose weight.

For example, vitamin A is needed to replace the cells that line the mouth and esophagus, and thiamin (vitamin B_1) is needed to maintain a normal appetite. Other vitamins, such as vitamin C and E, act as antioxidants in the body. They prevent or repair damage to cells due to oxidation (rusting) to help maintain your body tissues and prevent disease.

Minerals

Minerals are unlike any other nutrients in that they have an unequal number of electrons (negatively electrically charged particles) and protons (positively electrically charged particles) so they have either a positive or negative charge. The property of being electrically charged enables them to combine with other minerals to perform stable *complexes*. These complexes help you form things like bones, teeth, cartilage, and other tissues. The following are three important facts about minerals:

- They serve as the body's source of electrical power. You need electrical power in your body to do things like stimulate your muscles to contract, your heart to beat, and your nerves to carry nerve impulses.

- Humans require 15 minerals in order for their metabolisms to run well.

- You get minerals from a number of different foods. For example, calcium comes from dairy products but also from broccoli and dried beans. Phosphorus can be found in dairy products, but also in meats, seeds, and nuts.

DEFINITION

A **complex** is two individually charged atoms that bind together to form a neutral pair. For example, sodium and chloride bind together to make sodium chloride, also known as table salt.

The tendency of minerals to form complexes has some implication for their absorption from food. Calcium and zinc, for example, might combine with other minerals and supplements or with dietary fiber and form complexes that cannot be absorbed. Therefore, it's important to take calcium separate from other vitamins and minerals and at a time when you're not eating much fiber. The following is a list of required minerals:

- Calcium

- Chromium

- Copper

- Fluoride

- Iron

- Manganese

- Chloride

- Magnesium

- Molybdenum

- Phosphorus

- Iodine

- Potassium

- Selenium

- Sodium

- Zinc

Water

Water is one of the most important nutrients. In fact, adults' bodies are about 60 to 70 percent water by weight. Water provides the medium in which most chemical reactions take place in the body. It also plays important roles in metabolism, energy transformation, removal of toxins and wastes, and temperature regulation.

DID YOU KNOW?

If you're an adult woman, are in normal weather conditions, and have normal physical activity levels, you need to consume about 11 cups of water a day. If you're an adult male in similar circumstances, you need about 16 cups per day. Your need for water is even greater if you're in a hot, humid climate or have increased physical activity.

You should drink or otherwise take in enough water each day to replace the water you lose from perspiration, urination, and breathing. Most people don't realize that they lose a few liters of water each day and that they lose water every time they breathe.

Normally, you satisfy your need for water by drinking it and other fluids to satisfy your thirst. People generally get about 75 percent of their water intake from water and other fluids and about 2 percent from foods. You can tell that you have taken enough water if your urine is pale yellow, and you urinate a few times a day.

Proteins

Your body uses protein as a source of energy. However, protein's main function is to provide the body with amino acids, especially the essential amino acids, which it needs to build tissues such as muscles and bones. Remember, amino acids are the building blocks of proteins. You need eight amino acids to survive, but you must get them from the proteins that you take in.

Food sources of protein differ in quality, based on the types of amino acids they contain. The foods of high protein quality include all of the essential amino acids. Protein from milk, cheese, meat, eggs, fish, and other animal products is considered high quality. Plant sources of protein, with the exception of soybean, do not provide all of the essential amino acids.

DID YOU KNOW?

The word protein comes from the Greek word *proteus,* which means "of first importance."

You can combine plant foods such as grains or seeds with beans to create a high-quality protein. The amino acids found in each individual food complement each other to provide a source of complete protein. However, this is a little harder than getting your protein from meat, eggs, fish, and other animal products.

Fats

Fats are a concentrated source of energy. They are more satisfying to eat, so when you eat them, you actually take in fewer *calories* overall. Also, fats and proteins control your appetite better than carbohydrates, so eating some fat is a good thing for maintaining a healthy weight.

DEFINITION

A **calorie** is a unit of energy provided to the body by breaking down food into its component nutrients. Technically, it approximates the energy needed to increase the temperature of 1 gram of water by 1°C.

Fats perform a number of important functions in the body. They are the precursors for cholesterol and sex hormone synthesis, components of cell membranes, vehicles for carrying certain vitamins that are soluble in fat only, and suppliers of the essential fatty acids required for growth and health. As a matter of fact, 40 percent of your brain is made of fat!

There are different types of fat, and it's important to understand the differences. For example, essential fats are necessary for survival. If you don't get enough of them, or have the right ratios of them, you can become sick or die. On the other hand, trans fats have been linked to inflammation and other problems, and you're better off to eliminate them from your diet entirely.

DID YOU KNOW?

Low-fat diets are based on the idea that if you eat foods with less concentrated sources of energy and calories, you would not lose weight. However, no scientific evidence supports that these diets work.

To better understand fats, it's helpful to know a little bit about their chemical structure. Their names are tied to the structures. Fats come in different lengths and are divided into one of three categories: saturated, monounsaturated, and polyunsaturated.

The names of fats indicate how many, if any, double bonds occur in a particular fat. If the fat is saturated, it means no double bonds occur. If it's monounsaturated, it has one double bond, and polyunsaturated indicates many double bonds. This makes a big difference because the double bonds (also known as the saturation) and the length of the chain for the fat are what give the various fats their different properties. One of the reasons that the number of double bonds is important is because double bonds make the fat molecule more flexible.

The number of double bonds is also important because your cell membranes are made up of two layers of fatty acids connected to a "backbone." They are set up with the backbones on the outside of the double membrane and a fatty acid on the inside facing each other. You can imagine it as a lollipop with the candy being part of the backbone and the stick being the fatty acid. Therefore, an unsaturated fatty acid with no double bonds is not flexible and will look like the straight stick on a lollipop.

There is a branch of lollipops called "Safety Pops" and instead of using a stick, they use a piece of flexible string. The flexible string would be more like an unsaturated fatty acid because it has double bonds that make it more flexible. When you use the flexible fatty acids in a cell membrane, it makes it much more fluid and easier to transport nutrients and signals into the cell. Since you are what you eat, eating more unsaturated and polyunsaturated fats will give you more flexible cell membranes, which will allow for a better metabolism and a healthier body overall.

Cell Membrane

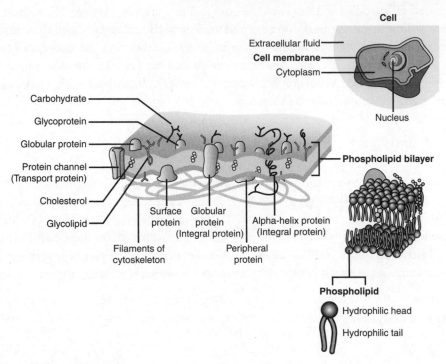

Diagram of a cell membrane.

THAT'S QUOTABLE

"Whether a fat is beneficial or harmful depends on its type, not how much you eat. This fact was confirmed by researchers at Harvard University who found no link between the percentage of daily calories consumed from fat and any disease including cancer, heart disease, and obesity."

—Christopher Cannon, M.D., and Elizabeth Vierck, M.S., *The Complete Idiot's Guide to the Anti-Inflammation Diet*

Fatty acids are usually bonded three at a time to a molecule called glycerol, which produces a molecule called a triglyceride. So when you have your blood work done and see elevated levels of triglycerides, you know that you have a lot of extra fatty acids floating around in your blood. Remember from Chapter 1 that oftentimes these extra fatty acids are created by eating extra sugar.

Saturated Fats

Saturated fats are fats with no double bonds. They are not flexible. They have generated a bad rap over the past 50 years and were initially thought to be the cause of cardiovascular disease and cancer. That being said, saturated fats are not all bad, and they might be helpful in some instances. It's a question of balance. For example, lauric acid, which is found in coconut oil, palm oil, and human breast milk, is an excellent fighter against viruses like HIV, chickenpox, and cytomegalovirus and has also been shown to help heal stomach irritation. Palmitic acid is found in palm oil, beef, eggs, milk, poultry, and seafood. It has been shown to be important in forming new memories and accessing old memories. Remember, your brain contains a lot of fat.

The bottom line with saturated fat is that, in moderation and without a significant intake of refined carbohydrates, it's pretty benign. It's important to remember that a diet with a high intake of saturated fats and high levels of insulin (due to sugar intake) can produce cholesterol particles that are easily oxidized and dangerous. When things are oxidized, it causes cell damage and inflammation, which can be a stressor on the body, creates an increased demand for cortisol, and leads to weight gain.

Unsaturated Fats

Monounsaturated fats contain one double bond and are more flexible than unsaturated fats. Oleic acid is found in olive oil, avocados, nuts, and some animal sources. These are the fats that the Mediterranean diet is based on. They are heart healthy and offer benefits such as improved insulin sensitivity, improved glucagon response, and decreased cholesterol levels. These types of fats are important in your diet.

Polyunsaturated fats contain many double bonds, and they are the most flexible overall. As it turns out, these are essential fats that you cannot make on your own, so you must get them from your diet. A key thing to appreciate is that if you don't get enough of these fats, or you don't get them in the right ratios, you can develop significant inflammation and illness. The two important subfamilies are the omega-3 family and the omega-6 family.

The omega-3 family comes from alpha linolenic acid (ALA), which is found in flax and other sources. Therefore, flax has the capability to create the more important omega-3s, EPA (eicosapentaenoic acid) and DHA (docosahexaenoic acid), but is not an efficient process. It's easier for people to take in their EPA and DHA from animal sources such as wild fish and game, flax-fed chicken eggs, and grass-fed meat. EPA is a potent anti-inflammatory and helps to thin the blood by reducing platelet stickiness, which reduces the risk of heart attack. DHA is critical for fetal breathing development and normal brain function throughout life. It's also anti-inflammatory. Bodies can interconvert EPA to DHA and back again; however, people function better if they take in enough of each of them.

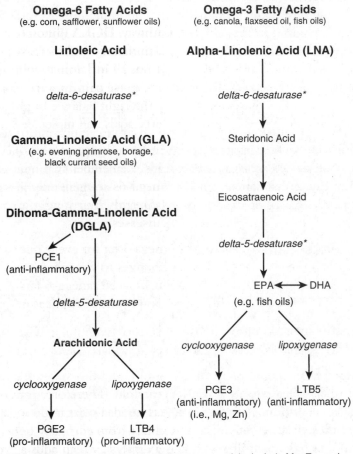

Diagram of an omega-3 and omega-6 pathway.

The omega-6 family is derived from linoleic acid (LA), which is found in high concentrations in vegetable oils such as safflower and sunflower. Linoleic acid and most of the other fatty acids it makes are pro-inflammatory. This creates irritation in the body and acts as a stressor, which creates a higher cortisol demand and the potential for subsequent weight gain.

Gamma linolenic acid (GLA) has one more double bond than linoleic acid and comes from borage, primrose, and hemp oils. The interesting thing about GLA is that it is the only anti-inflammatory metabolite in the omega-6 pathway because it can block the production of inflammatory prostaglandins. GLA production is reduced with high levels of insulin and with viral infection, so in those instances, more inflammation occurs.

The last two metabolites in the omega-6 pathway, DGLA (dihomo-gamma-linolenic acid) and AA (arachidonic acid), are pro-inflammatory and increase production of inflammatory molecules. Keep in mind that not all inflammation is bad. You need it to help fight off bacterial and viral invaders, cause pain to warn of injury, and generally protect you. You just need to have the right balance in place between your pro-inflammatory and anti-inflammatory fatty acids and molecules.

A major problem with your current diet is that you have a significant imbalance between the omega-3 and omega-6 fatty acids. Remember that omega-3s are generally thought of as anti-inflammatory and omega-6s are generally pro-inflammatory. The ratio between omega-3s and omega-6s controls your weight, elements of cancer, Parkinson's, Alzheimer's, and several other diseases.

Originally, your diet provided about one omega-3 fat for every one to three omega-6 fats. Because of all the corn oils and other changes to your diet, your current ratio is believed to be one omega-3 fat to between 10 to 20 omega-6 fats. You can see that this tips the scale in favor of inflammation and is one of the reasons people have an increase in chronic disease.

Trans Fats

The concept of trans fats is only about 50 years old. Therefore, your metabolism, which was designed millions of years ago, has no idea what to do with a trans fat. Trans fats are created when polyunsaturated fats from corn, soy beans, and similar oils are exposed to heat, hydrogen gas, and a catalyst, which adds a hydrogen onto the polyunsaturated fat. Essentially, this gets rid of the double bonds and makes the fat look saturated. The good news for the food industry is that these fats are solid or semisolid at room temperature, and they don't go rancid quickly, so products have a longer shelf life. The problem is that trans fats damage your liver function, cause problems with your blood lipid levels, and destroy your sensitivity to insulin. These are all significant contributors to weight gain and obesity.

THAT'S QUOTABLE

"… suffice it to say that trans fatty acids are b-a-a-a-d. They raise your total blood cholesterol level and your LDL or bad cholesterol; lower your HDL or good cholesterol; and are suspected of contributing to obesity and diabetes."

—Robert L. Wolke (www.professorscience.com), Professor Emeritus of Chemistry at the University of Pittsburgh

Trans fats are seen in many packaged convenience foods and fast foods such as cookies, french fries, fried chicken, biscuits, fried fish sandwiches, donuts, muffins, crackers, and many other things. According to the findings by the Institute of Medicine, "it is recommended that trans-fatty acids consumption be as low as possible while consuming a nutritionally adequate diet." Dr. Jeffrey Aron of the University of California at San Francisco states, "There should be a warning label on food made with this stuff like there is with nicotine. It is that bad for you."

New research from the Harvard Nurses' Health study shows that trans-fatty acids are linked to an increase in inflammation throughout the body, especially in women who are already overweight. Large increases in risk of heart disease occur with as little as 3 to 4 grams of trans-fatty acids daily. Even if something only has half a gram of trans fat on the label per serving, if you eat a lot of processed food throughout the day, those half grams of trans fats per serving could add up to the 3 to 4 grams that would put you at risk.

THAT'S QUOTABLE

"By our most conservative estimates, replacement of partially hydrogenated fat in the U.S. diet with natural unhydrogenated vegetable oils would prevent approximately 30,000 premature coronary deaths per year, and epidemiologic evidence suggests this number is closer to 100,000 premature deaths annually."

—Harvard School of Public Health

Carbohydrates

Carbohydrates are the molecules carbon, hydrogen, and oxygen that are used as a source of energy for the bodies. They can be simple (glucose) or complex (many glucose molecules attached together). Plant sources are naturally occurring complex carbohydrates that contain nutrients and fiber. Carbohydrates include a wide range of food types, including refined and undefined breads and cereals, vegetables, fruits, and legumes. Vegetables, fruits, legumes, and refined grains are considered more favorable because they tend to convert to sugar more slowly and are more slowly absorbed into the bloodstream.

In addition to balancing insulin, these "good carbs" increase glucagon, support thyroid health, and optimize the production of sex hormones and DHEA. These things can all lead to weight loss. Refined carbohydrates such as white rice, pasta, and all forms of sugar do not have any significant nutritional value and are rapidly absorbed as sugar into the bloodstream. This raises the blood sugar and creates a large demand for insulin, which you know can lead to insulin resistance and fat storage.

Glycemic Index

The speed with which carbohydrates are converted into blood sugar is one of the determinants for whether or not a food promotes hormone balance or imbalance and whether the food increases or decreases the risk for disease. The glycemic index (GI) is a system of measuring the conversion speed of individual carbohydrate foods and the rate at which they increase your blood sugar. It was originally developed in 1979 by scientists at the University of Toronto and Oxford University in England to help diabetics make better food choices. Since then, scientists at the University of Sydney in Australia have carried out a significant amount of research on the subject and have established an international database of foods and their GI rankings at www. glycemicindex.com.

THAT'S QUOTABLE

"Believe me, sugar is the devil. It's here to ruin you. A diet based on white bread, white rice, cereals, soda, and low-fat products is loaded with sugar."

—Michael Aziz, M.D., *The Perfect Ten Diet*

The index ranks foods according to how quickly the human body converts the carbohydrate in the food into glucose in the blood. The more rapidly a food is absorbed and converts to glucose, the faster and higher it raises the level of blood glucose. Based on research for individual foods, each food is assigned a numerical GI rating from 0 to 100, based on its impact on blood sugar. Pure glucose, as a food, is given a value of 100 and used as a reference point. It should be noted that the index is used only for foods that contain a significant amount of carbohydrates.

To make it easier to use the glycemic index, foods are generally grouped into low, medium, and high GI rankings. Low GI foods do the best job of keeping blood sugar level stable, but that doesn't mean you can never eat foods with a higher GI ranking. The glycemic indexes for some popular foods are as follows:

- Most vegetables are almost 0 GI.

- Root vegetables except potatoes are usually low to medium GI.

- Potatoes generally have a high GI.

- Fruits from northern and Mediterranean climates are low GI.

- Fruits from tropical climates tend to be medium GI.

- White and whole-wheat breads are both high GI in any form.

- Sourdough breads have a low GI because acidity slows down digestion.

- Dense breads made with whole grains other than wheat and dough made with spelt flour have a low or medium GI.

- Acidic ingredients, such as balsamic vinegar used to dip bread, will reduce the GI.

- Nuts and seeds are low GI.

- Brown and white rice are high GI.

- Basmati rice is medium GI.

- Quinoa and pearled barley are low GI.

- Sweetened sodas and sugary drinks are high GI.

- Beans and legumes, such as lentils and peas, are very low GI.

Glycemic Load

The glycemic load is probably even more meaningful for weight control than the glycemic index. The glycemic load measures the real response of your blood sugar—and therefore, your insulin level—to an entire meal. Because the glycemic load is the effect of the total meal on your blood sugar, it isn't related only to the original amount of carbohydrate.

Many factors determine how quickly carbohydrates turn into sugar in your body. These include the type of carbohydrate (low, medium, or high GI carb) and the amount of protein, fat, and fiber you eat at the same time as well. If you eat a number of foods that have high GIs and don't include anything to slow down the absorption of the sugar (like proteins or fats), you will have a high glycemic load meal. That means that there will be a large amount of sugar rapidly entering the bloodstream, which will require the production of a large amount of insulin to process it.

Low glycemic load meals have combinations of food containing mainly low glycemic index carbohydrates or added protein, fat, and fiber that slow the absorption of the sugar. Therefore, if your meal has a low glycemic load, you do not have a rapid rise in blood sugar, and you do not need to produce a lot of insulin to process the smaller amount of blood sugar.

To give you an idea of how glycemic load works, consider the following examples. The first example is pasta with marinara sauce and Italian bread for dinner followed by chocolate cake for dessert. This dinner has a high glycemic load. The pasta, Italian bread, and chocolate cake are all high GI foods. Therefore, they turn into sugar very quickly, raise your blood sugar, and create a high demand for insulin. There is no fiber, protein, or fat in the meal to slow the absorption of the sugars from the carbohydrate.

To help lower the glycemic load of this dinner, reduce the amount of pasta and add meat to the sauce. Also, the Italian bread can be changed to sourdough bread dipped in oil and vinegar. It would also help to add more vegetables, green beans, and garlic sautéed in olive oil or a salad with mixed greens and raw vegetables drizzled in olive oil and balsamic vinegar. The dessert can be changed from chocolate cake to mixed berries with nuts and whipped cream.

You can see how the addition of the meat increases the protein, which slows down the absorption of the sugars in the pasta. In addition, sourdough bread has a lower GI than Italian bread. Dipping it into the vinegar adds acidity, which slows down the absorption; dipping it into the olive oil adds fat, which also slows down absorption. Last, adding the sautéed green beans and mixed berries with nuts increases the fiber and the nutrients in the meal. At the end of the day, the second meal sounds delicious, too, but the sugars from the pasta and bread will be absorbed much more slowly and not cause as much of a spike in blood sugar.

Grains

Whole grains contain all the essential parts of the grain's seed, along with its nutrients. In their natural state growing in the fields, whole grains are the entire seed of the plant. The grain is made up of three parts: bran, germ, and endosperm.

- The bran is the outer covering of the grain, and it contains antioxidants, B vitamins, and fiber.

- The germ is the embryo, which can sprout into a new plant. It contains many B vitamins, some protein, minerals, and healthy fats.

- The endosperm is the germ's food supply. It supplies energy to the young plant so it can grow and is the largest portion of the kernel. It contains starchy carbohydrates, proteins, and small amounts of vitamins and minerals.

Although whole grains contain all three parts, refined grains only have the endosperm, which contains the starchy carbohydrates and some protein. Without the bran and germ, about one quarter of the grain's protein is lost, along with key nutrients.

Examples of generally accepted whole-grain foods and flours are amaranth, barley, colored and brown rice, buckwheat, bulgur, corn and whole cornmeal, kamut, millet, oatmeal and whole oats, popcorn, quinoa, sorghum, spelt, whole rye, whole or cracked wheat, wheat berries, and wild rice. If you see the words "whole grain" on a food label, the product is required by the federal government to have virtually the same proportions of bran, germ, and endosperm as the harvested kernel does before it's processed. Some foods that you might think are whole grains actually are not. For instance, soybean products and other beans and sunflower seeds and roots such as arrowroot do not meet the FDA's definition of the whole grain.

Vegetables

Vegetables are a source of carbohydrates that contain large amounts of vitamins, minerals, phytonutrients, and fiber. It's the fiber in the vegetables that slows down the absorption of the carbohydrates so your blood sugar does not go up and you don't have an increased demand for insulin. Vegetables that are raw, mildly steamed, or stir-fried maintain most of their fiber. Starchy vegetables such as white potatoes, carrots (especially cooked), and beets don't have as much fiber so they might cause an increase in blood sugar if they are eaten in large quantities without any other source of fiber, protein, or fat.

If you're trying to lose weight, or not exercising regularly, limit the quantities of these starchy vegetables until you have better insulin balance. However, you can eat many vegetables in unlimited quantities. Cruciferous vegetables like broccoli and cauliflower contain a substance called indole-3-carbinol, which is important in the metabolism of estrogen for men and women.

Legumes

Legumes, or beans, are excellent carbohydrates and also contain small amounts of protein. Include kidney beans, navy beans, lentils, black beans, and garbanzo beans in your diet because they are high in soluble fiber, have a low GI, and do not rapidly raise the blood sugar or create a high insulin demand. They are also an excellent source of antioxidants. Antioxidants help to fight free radicals, or oxidation, which can create cell damage and inflammation in your body. You can include legumes in your diet in many ways, such as in salads, chili, hummus, and other great dishes.

Fruits

Fruits are important carbohydrates because they are high in vitamins, minerals, fiber, enzymes, and water. The sugar in fruits is fructose, which is not to be confused with high fructose corn syrup. The fiber in the fruits slows down the absorption of the fructose sugar so it does not negatively impact insulin levels. That being said, fruit juices do not contain fiber, so the sugar in the fruit juice will rapidly enter the bloodstream, raise your blood sugar, and create high insulin demand. Therefore, you should eat whole fruits rather than drink fruit juices.

The fruits with the lowest GI include berries, cherries, melons, oranges, apples, pears, and grapes. Fruits like mangoes and bananas have less fiber and might be more likely to raise your blood sugar, so they should be eaten in moderation.

Fiber

Fiber is the indigestible part of fruits, whole grains, legumes, and vegetables. It's an important part of your diet because it can make you feel full while limiting the number of calories you eat. Fiber slows the absorption of sugars from your digestive tract to your bloodstream. It also helps you feel full and provides bulk in your intestines so the waste moves through them more easily. Grains vary greatly in the amount of fiber they contain, ranging from 3.5 percent in rice to 15 percent in barley and bulgur. Many of the refined grains have the fiber refined out of them. For example, 100 grams of whole-grain wheat flour has 12.2 grams of fiber while white, bleached, all-purpose flour only has 2.7 grams of fiber.

Fiber is a powerful substance that has the capability to help you lose weight; lower your blood sugar and cholesterol; and reduce the risk of cancer, heart disease, diabetes, and inflammation. It's like a sponge that helps to soak up the fat and sugar in your intestines and slows down, and actually inhibits, some of their absorption. Therefore, you have less of a spike in your blood sugar and less of a demand for insulin. Your body has to work harder to digest foods with a lot of fiber. Consider the difference between eating an apple and drinking a glass of apple juice. They contain the same basic nutrients, but because the apple has so much more fiber, it needs more time to break down and takes more energy to do it. The apple has a lower GI because it does not affect the blood sugar as much as apple juice would. Fiber is one of the major things that determine the glycemic load of the meal.

The Least You Need to Know

- Poor food choices send the wrong messages to your hormones and genes, which control your cells.
- Drink or otherwise take in enough water each day to replace the water you lose from perspiration, urination, and breathing.
- Saturated fats are helpful in some instances.
- Unsaturated fats are heart healthy.
- The speed with which carbohydrates are converted into blood sugar is one of the determinants for whether or not a food promotes hormone balance or imbalance.
- If a meal has a low glycemic load, you will not have a rapid rise in blood sugar, and you will not need to produce a lot of insulin to handle it.

Principle #3: Enhance Your Hormonal Balance

In This Chapter

- How unbalanced hormones can make you fat
- Bioidentical versus synthetic hormones
- The safety of bioidentical hormones
- Hormone testing
- Questions to ask your physician

Your hormones maintain a very intricate balance within your body. This chapter explains how having unbalanced hormones can affect your weight and your general health. It also discusses the difference between bioidentical and synthetic hormones and the options available to you for testing your hormone levels. This chapter clarifies why if you need hormone therapy, it is important to take bioidentical hormones. Finally, this chapter provides guidelines for choosing a physician who is knowledgeable about hormones and has a holistic approach to medical care.

Susan's Story

Susan is a pleasantly plump 42-year-old schoolteacher. She came to me complaining that her plumpness had turned into obesity with a weight gain of 20 pounds. She also was increasingly fatigued. She was losing her hair, her breasts were tender, and her menstrual periods were irregular. Susan's symptoms increased over the past year. She had gained weight, added belly fat around her middle, and had difficulty falling asleep. By the time Susan came to see me, it was taking her one to two hours to fall asleep at night.

Before becoming my patient, she didn't take time for breakfast, and she often grabbed a sandwich and soda at the school cafeteria for lunch. In the evening, she had papers to correct and lesson plans to complete, so with little time to cook, she ate take-out food most nights.

After taking Susan's diet and health history, I looked at her lab work. It showed that her hormone levels were awry: her progesterone level was low, her thyroid was not functioning well, and her cortisol levels were elevated, which is a sign of persistent stress.

What was going on with Susan? Her high stress levels were creating a large demand for cortisol. In order to meet that demand, her body was using up progesterone. The high cortisol was causing her to put on belly fat and made it difficult for her to fall asleep. Her low progesterone created an imbalance with estrogen, which led to irregular menstrual periods and breast tenderness. Because of her high cortisol levels, her body was on alert for significant stress and shut down her thyroid because it thought it needed to conserve energy. Her low thyroid levels contributed to weight gain, fatigue, dry skin, dry hair and hair loss, and constipation.

My prescription for Susan was to switch her diet to whole foods and eliminate all refined carbohydrates. I also encouraged her to eat regularly (every three hours) to maintain a steady blood sugar and reduce her cortisol demand. I reviewed some stress management techniques with her such as deep breathing, gratitude, and yoga. (I describe those techniques and many more in Chapter 16.) Because of her significant symptoms, I started her on bioidentical progesterone to support her menstrual cycle and on bioidentical thyroid replacement.

Susan slowly started to get her life back. She is able to sleep better, and her fatigue has improved. By setting boundaries at her job, she is able to find more time at home to prepare healthy, nutritious foods. She joined a community gym and is taking a fitness class twice a week, which is further reducing her stress levels. Over the course of three months, she has lost 20 pounds and regained her energy.

This chapter looks at some of Susan's issues and how you can learn from her story.

How Having Unbalanced Hormones Can Affect Your Weight

Unbalanced hormones can affect your weight in several ways. As you saw in Chapter 2, many major hormones are derived from cholesterol, including your stress hormone, cortisol, and your sex hormones, estrogen and testosterone. The best way to maintain hormone balance is to eat appropriately, get enough sleep, exercise, eliminate toxins, and reduce your stress levels. However, hormones can be so far out of balance that these measures are not enough to reverse the problem. This is more likely to happen if you are over 40 because your hormone levels naturally decline after this age.

As the restorative hormones begin to decline, an imbalance becomes harmful. For example, in men, it is known that low testosterone contributes to heart disease, diabetes, osteoporosis, and depression. In women, an imbalance of estrogen and progesterone can lead to symptoms such as weight gain, fatigue, mood changes, insomnia, and difficulty concentrating.

Often, high levels of stress, poor diet, lack of sleep, and lack of exercise make midlife hormone depletion worse. This combination creates problems such as fatigue, weight gain, depression, diabetes, high cholesterol, irritable bowel, and sleep disturbances. These symptoms often send people to their physician. If the physician gives the patient a prescription to treat the symptoms without treating the underlying hormone imbalance, the situation can spiral out of control.

I've had patients who visited doctors to treat one or more of the previous symptoms. Instead of treating the root of the problem, hormone imbalance, the doctor gave them prescriptions to cover the symptoms. Because they still had their initial imbalance, they developed other symptoms and got other prescriptions; then they developed a side effect from one of the prescriptions and so got yet another prescription, and so on. By the time I met them, they were taking six or seven different prescriptions.

Cortisol Demand

Pregnenolone and progesterone, the first two hormones to come from cholesterol, have the choice to make either cortisol or your sex hormones. So the first thing that can create weight gain with hormone imbalance is having a high demand for cortisol because you start shunting your building blocks to make cortisol instead of your sex hormones.

This is important, because estrogen and testosterone help build up the body. As a matter of fact, estrogen has more than 400 functions, including increasing your metabolic rate, improving insulin sensitivity, helping to maintain muscle, helping you sleep deeply, enhancing energy, improving mood, and helping with the formation of neurotransmitters in your brain. Of note, estrogen helps men as well.

DID YOU KNOW?

In men, estrogen is important for sexual desire and heart health. However, they don't need too much. Because testosterone is converted estrogen due to enzymes in belly fat, if they have a large amount of belly fat, they can make too much estrogen and have symptoms such as erectile dysfunction, breast enlargement, and prostate enlargement.

Perimenopause

In the years leading up to menopause (called *perimenopause*), women start having hormone fluctuations, starting with lower progesterone. This is because they are not regularly releasing eggs and are not producing enough progesterone as a result of it. If you're in this group and you're also stressed, your progesterone will be even lower because your body will be busy using it as a building block to help make cortisol. This is why women might notice an increase in symptoms when they're under stress.

As you get closer to *menopause*, and your estrogen level finally begins to fall significantly, you might notice even more of an increase in fat around your belly. This happens because some of estrogen's functions are to increase metabolism and insulin sensitivity. As perimenopause and menopause progress, symptoms might increase, including hot flashes, night sweats, difficulty sleeping, weight gain, poor memory, mood swings, irregular bleeding, and a host of other problems. Some women can relieve the symptoms with lifestyle changes, supplements, and herbs. However, some women choose to replace the missing hormones with hormone replacement therapy.

> **DEFINITION**
>
> **Perimenopause** is a time when ovarian function starts to decline, eggs are not regularly released, and hormone imbalances like low progesterone start to occur. The hormone imbalances can cause symptoms like hot flashes, night sweats, irregular menses, difficulty sleeping, and many others. It can last for years prior to menopause.
>
> **Menopause** is the lack of menses for 12 continuous months due to ovarian failure. Estrogen levels go down for many (but not all) women at this time.

Testosterone

Testosterone is another hormone that helps build up your body. In addition, testosterone increases the sense of well-being, increases muscle mass and strength, helps maintain memory, decreases excess body fat, enhances libido, and helps maintain bone strength. It's easy to see how you can gain weight if you don't have enough of these hormones. Also, because chronically high levels of cortisol cause an increase of belly fat, you're on a path in which you gain weight and have fewer ways to get rid of it.

If you're a man and you think that you can "tune out" during the discussions of hormone therapy, you're wrong! Because of high stress levels, inadequate sleep, poor diet, and toxin exposure, many men suffer from low testosterone. As a matter of fact, studies show that a population-wide decrease has occurred in overall testosterone levels in men of all ages. One in five men under the age of 40 have testosterone levels that are low for their ages. It is staggering to think that 20 percent of younger men can have symptoms of low testosterone.

The symptoms of low testosterone include depression, weight gain, difficulty sleeping, low libido, erectile dysfunction, and fatigue. Low testosterone can also contribute to a number of diseases such as heart disease, diabetes, osteoporosis, and Alzheimer's. Many men go to their physicians with symptoms of low testosterone and are given medications to address their various complaints, such as depression, difficulty sleeping, and erectile dysfunction. Because these medications don't deal with the source of the problem, low testosterone, the symptoms eventually get worse, and these men are prescribed even more medication.

Because testosterone is instrumental in helping to build lean muscle mass, low testosterone contributes to increased fat mass and weight gain. This sets off a chain of events that often lead to fatigue, depression, inflammation, and further weight gain.

Stress

Imbalance of cortisol and the sex hormones is not the only way to gain weight. Often, when people are under stress and have a high cortisol demand, they crave sugars and refined carbohydrates. This craving, combined with the fact that high cortisol also causes higher blood sugar, creates an imbalance with insulin. Insulin is the hormone that helps handle blood sugar levels. If too much insulin is present in the body because you have so much sugar to deal with from your diet, your body eventually stops listening to the insulin, and you start to store all the sugar as fat rather than use it for energy. Insulin resistance also creates high blood pressure and high cholesterol.

Thyroid

Another issue with weight gain due to hormone imbalance concerns the thyroid. The thyroid gland, located in the front of the neck, secretes thyroid hormone, which is in charge of the metabolism. The amount of thyroid hormone and level of metabolism is closely tied to the overall hormone balance. If your cortisol level is high, the body thinks that you're in a crisis and that you'll need to conserve your energy to handle the crisis. Therefore, it tells your thyroid to secrete less active hormone and reduce your metabolism so that you can conserve energy. Your thyroid gland activity is also closely tied to levels of other hormones like estrogen.

What Are Bioidentical Hormones?

Bioidentical hormones like estradiol (E2) and progesterone are often in the news. However, a major problem exists with the current studies on hormones reported by the media: they do not distinguish between bioidentical and nonbioidentical hormones for the following three major reasons:

- Physicians usually don't receive training in bioidentical hormone therapy during medical school.

- Because bioidentical hormones are identical in structure to the hormones made by the body, they cannot be patented. Therefore, pharmaceutical companies are not as interested in developing them as medications. However, they can (and do) develop unique delivery systems like patches and gels.

- Many physicians are so busy taking care of their day-to-day practices that they don't have time to do the extra learning required to adequately treat patients with bioidentical hormone therapy. Also, many physicians get their information from the media and pharmaceutical reps, so they are influenced by what they hear and are not presented with all of the options.

Bioidentical hormones have the same shape and structure as those your body naturally makes. Because they have the same chemical structure, they have the correct shape to fit into all of the receptors on the cells in your body. Therefore, they can command your cells to do all the things that they're supposed to do.

What is interesting is that physicians use pharmaceutical bioidentical hormones all the time, and no one makes a fuss. The insulin and thyroid hormones that are routinely prescribed by physicians are bioidentical to human hormones. It seems that the confusion only arises when we're talking about E2 (an estrogen) and progesterone.

Hormones and receptors are often compared to a lock and key. The hormone is the key, and the receptor on the cell is the lock. If even one small difference exists in the key, it won't fit into the lock. In order for the cells in particular parts of your body—such as your brain, heart, breast, and fat—to work, the hormone must be a perfect fit to the receptor. If it's not a perfect fit, the instructions will be garbled.

More importantly, bioidentical hormones are broken down (metabolized) the same way your body naturally breaks down hormones. This is critical because if your body does not know how to metabolize a substance, the result is an imbalance. The bottom line is that, ideally, you want to have hormones in your body that are the same as those it makes naturally.

Many types of biochemical hormones are available, including estrogen, progesterone, testosterone, thyroid, DHEA, and cortisol. These hormones are available commercially as well as through compounded pharmacies.

What Are Nonbioidentical Hormones?

Most of the research reported in the news is not about bioidentical hormones. The nonbioidentical hormones (synthetic) that are usually studied are natural hormones that have had their structures slightly changed so that the manufacturer can patent them.

Think about the lock and key analogy. Synthetic hormones have had their keys changed so they won't fit into the lock as well, if at all. This means that you won't get the effects you are expecting.

The following two synthetic hormones are prescribed for women in or near menopause:

- Premarin, one of the most widely known nonbioidentical estrogens, contains horse estrogens known as equelin and equilenin instead of estrogen, which do not react in your body like your own estrogen does. On top of that, your natural estrogen is metabolized in a few hours, but horse estrogen can stay in your body for up to 13 weeks!

- Provera, a progestin (not progesterone), is different than the natural hormone that women produce when they are younger. Your natural progesterone balances estrogen, lowers cholesterol, helps your body eliminate fats, and has a natural calming effect. Provera, or medroxyprogesterone acetate, stops the protective effects of estrogen on your heart and has other side effects, including weight gain and fluid retention. It's amazing what a few extra side chains on a molecule can do to change the way it acts in your body!

Safety Comparison Between Bioidentical and Nonbioidentical Hormones

I am often asked whether taking hormones such as Premarin and Provera is safe. Many physicians answer this question by quoting the government-sponsored Women's Health Initiative study, which was widely covered by the media in 2002. In the study, government researchers used Premarin and Provera as representative of hormone replacement therapy. Their goal was to study its effects on heart disease, bone health, breast cancer, dementia, and other age-related issues. Interestingly, they didn't look at the most important thing to midlife women: relief of menopausal symptoms. In fact, most women request hormone replacement therapy to treat night sweats, insomnia, and the other problems that occur during menopause.

In July 2002, the researchers stopped the Premarin and Provera combined arm of the study because the risk of breast cancer was significantly high. However, this finding does not apply to all hormones, and certainly not to bioidentical hormones.

As I mentioned earlier in this chapter, Premarin, or horse estrogen, stays in your body for 13 weeks. Provera is known to create abnormal cell divisions in breast tissue, which increases the risk of breast cancer. Also, the use of progestins such as Provera interferes with your body's own production of natural progesterone, so you have even less of its good effects.

DID YOU KNOW?

One study of 54,000 postmenopausal women in France compared the risk of breast cancer among women using hormone replacement therapy, such as Premarin and Provera, or bioidentical hormone therapy. Risk for breast cancer increased by up to 70 percent among those women taking progestins such as Provera compared to those taking bioidentical progesterone.

Do You Need Hormone Therapy?

The decision to take hormone replacement therapy should be made with your physician. In this world of "one size fits all" medications to treat symptoms, hormone replacement therapy should be customized to you, with an understanding of your genetic, environmental, and physiologic risk factors.

TRUSTY TIP

If you start bioidentical hormone replacement therapy, remember that your relationship with your doctor is not just about using hormones. You and your physician are a team, working together to optimize your diet and maintain a lifestyle that will keep your hormone levels balanced.

In her book *HRT: The Answers*, Dr. Pamela Smith discusses five main reasons you should consider natural hormone replacement therapy: relief of menopausal symptoms, prevention of memory loss, heart health, prevention of osteoporosis, and general tissue growth and repair. I have seen a number of significant symptoms occur in women (and men) as their hormone levels declined either due to aging or poor lifestyle choices.

It's important to understand that this situation can and should be reversed in order to maintain optimal health and brain function. Since bioidentical hormones act the same way that your naturally produced hormones would act in your body, they're an excellent way to replenish those hormones. Of course, proper diet and lifestyle choices play a key role as well.

Hormone Testing

If you are considering hormone replacement therapy, you should have your hormone levels tested so that you can make an informed decision. It's important to locate a physician who understands bioidentical hormone therapy and can treat you in a holistic fashion. See Appendix B to find physicians that practice this way.

A number of different ways to test hormone levels are available. Many physicians are familiar with serum or blood testing. This type of testing is an excellent way to look at a number of hormones, especially thyroid hormones and insulin. Serum testing is used to look at hormones such as estrogen, progesterone, testosterone, and DHEA. However, serum tests look at the total amount of the hormones in your blood, whether they are free for use by your body or bound to a storage protein. Ask your doctor to request a free hormone fraction test separately so you can see how much free (active) hormone you have available.

Saliva tests look at free hormone levels, which are the unbound hormones "free and available" for your body to use. It's also the best way to measure your adrenal cortisol production at different points throughout the day. You can also use saliva testing for other hormones such as estrogen, progesterone, testosterone, DHEA, and melatonin. This type of testing can be convenient because you can collect a saliva sample at home and send it to the lab yourself.

Urine testing is helpful to determine the various levels of hormones in your system, especially estrogen, progesterone, DHEA, growth hormone, and cortisol.

Urine testing is also used to look at the way your hormones are metabolized. Estrogen metabolism is important in determining your risk for breast cancer. (Two women can take the same amount of estrogen, and if one metabolizes her estrogen in a healthier fashion, her risk of breast cancer is lower.) Many things contribute to a healthy metabolism, including your genes, your diet, the amount of sleep you get, and many other lifestyle factors.

Questions to Ask Your Physician

If you're considering hormone replacement therapy, it's important to see a physician who is trained in bioidentical hormone therapy and has a holistic approach to medicine. Ask potential doctors the following questions:

- **Have you had training in bioidentical hormone therapy?** Although more physicians are being trained in the importance of bioidentical hormone therapy, most don't understand the difference between Premarin and Provera and natural bioidentical estrogen and progesterone. It's important that you use only bioidentical hormones as a way to balance your system and enhance your overall health. Physicians who have training in bioidentical hormone replacement therapy will understand how to customize your hormones and how to use the many delivery systems that are available, including tablets, creams, gels, lozenges, patches, and many other forms.

- **Do you know about the different types of hormone testing available?** It's important for your physician to understand that the type of testing you require depends on what hormones you're looking at and what kind of therapy you are using.

- **Will you test my adrenal glands?** A strong relationship exists between the adrenal glands, which produce the stress hormone cortisol, and many other hormones in your body. Your adrenal glands can become fatigued if they have been working to produce cortisol for a long period of time, and they can no longer meet the demand. Therefore, it's important to know how they're functioning so you can take steps to heal them if you need to.

The Least You Need to Know

- The studies on hormones currently reported by the media do not distinguish between bioidentical and nonbioidentical hormones.
- Because they have the same chemical structure, bioidentical hormones have the correct shape to fit into all of the receptors on the cells in your body.
- If you are considering hormone replacement therapy, you should have your hormone levels tested first so that you can make an informed decision.
- It's important to work with a physician who understands bioidentical hormone therapy and can treat you in a holistic fashion.

Principle #4: Energize!

In This Chapter

- How stress causes the release of cortisol
- How stress can make you fat
- Stress and adrenal fatigue
- Sleep deprivation and weight gain

Lowering your stress level will allow you to get to and maintain a healthy weight. This chapter addresses the effects of stress and how to overcome it.

Julie's Story

Julie is a 32-year-old emergency room nurse who came to see me with exhaustion, asthma, difficulty concentrating, and weight gain. She has worked in an emergency room for the past three years on the night shift. She enjoys her job and loves excitement. As a matter of fact, she states that she has always been an "adrenaline junkie." She does four shifts a week from 11 P.M. to 7 A.M. and is busy for the entire time. She usually does not have time to eat anything except for the cookies and candies that sit on the counter at the nurses' station. When she gets home in the morning, she takes her two children to school at 8:30 A.M. Then she goes home and does housework before she tries to lie down around 10 A.M. She tries to sleep until the children come home around 3 P.M. and gets up to help them with their schoolwork, do some more housework, and make dinner for her husband and children.

On nights that Julie works, she tries to take a quick nap in the evening before she goes back to work. If she is not working, she stays up with her husband until about 11 P.M. Often, on nights when she doesn't have to work, she still finds it difficult to sleep through the night. She wakes up once or twice and goes downstairs to get a snack. However, when it's time to wake up in the morning, she is exhausted and needs to hit the snooze alarm four or five times before she gets up out of bed. It is getting harder and harder for her to continue working and taking care of the children. Last week, she ended up as a patient in the emergency room with an asthma attack. For Julie, this was a blast from the past; she had asthma as a child but had not had an attack in years.

Julie's shift work and inadequate rest after her shift were creating a significant hormone imbalance. Disrupted sleep patterns can cause an imbalance in cortisol, insulin, growth hormone, and hormones connected to appetite (leptin and ghrelin).

When I tested Julie's hormones, I found that her cortisol levels were very low throughout the day and elevated in the evening, her blood sugar and cholesterol were elevated, and she had signs of inflammation. This combination of lab tests suggested insulin resistance and adrenal fatigue. (I cover adrenal fatigue in Chapter 16.) It usually occurs after a long period of chronic stress and high cortisol demand that wears out the adrenal gland, which can't meet the body's demand for cortisol. Once someone has adrenal fatigue, it is difficult for them to reduce inflammation and they are more likely to develop problems like asthma and allergies. This is what happened in Julie's case.

In order to treat Julie, we needed to improve her sleep patterns and her eating habits. I encouraged her to stop eating processed foods and refined carbohydrates. I also told her that she needed to eat every two to three hours while she was awake and make sure her small meals and snacks consisted of proteins, vegetables, and healthy fats. Julie learned the importance of preparing batches of whole foods in advance so she would have healthy choices available to take to work with her.

Julie and her husband were concerned about her health, especially in light of the recent asthma attack. When I told her how important it was for her to get sleep after her shift, they made the decision to hire someone part time to take the children to school and do some basic housework in the morning so Julie could go right to bed when she got home. She was instructed to make the room as dark and quiet as possible and to try to sleep for seven hours when she got home. She also used some supplements to help stabilize her adrenals. Although it took Julie a while to get adjusted to her new routine, eventually her sleep patterns improved, and she had a lot more energy. Over the next five months, she lost 15 of the 30 pounds she had gained and did not have another asthma attack.

This chapter looks at some of the reasons you need to get more sleep and reduce your stress to avoid symptoms like Julie's.

Stress Everywhere!

The word *stress* has many different meanings. In fact, Dictionary.com lists 14 different definitions, and *Merriam Webster* lists 12. It's a universal word and has been adopted in many languages, including Japanese, Hindi, and French.

Medically speaking, I think of stress as a specific response by bodies to fear, pain, or another stimulus, which disturbs or interferes with your normal physiological equilibrium. Its importance is in what it means to the person experiencing the stress. How you feel in response to a stressor controls your physical response. In addition, getting adequate sleep is important for reducing stress and losing weight.

 THAT'S QUOTABLE

"Stress is difficult for scientists to define because it is a subjective sensation associated with varied symptoms that differ for each of us. In addition, stress is not always a synonym for distress. Situations like a steep roller coaster ride that cause fear and anxiety for some can prove highly pleasurable for others. Winning a race or election may be more stressful than losing, but this is good stress."

—Paul J. Rosch, M.D., F.A.C.P.; President, The American Institute of Stress; Clinical Professor of Medicine and Psychiatry, New York Medical College

Common stress reactions are feelings of anxiety, heart palpitations, and stomach ache. Far too often, these responses cause emotional and physical overload. External events and internal responses to them exhaust your ability to cope, which causes fatigue, mood changes, difficulty concentrating, and disease. It can eventually cause you to gain weight.

The three most common sources of stress in your body are mental and emotional stress, chronic inflammation, and blood sugar imbalance. Many different factors can contribute to and are amplified by your response to stress, such as fear, anxiety, depression, feelings of helplessness, pain syndromes, infection, inflammation, low blood sugar, inadequate sleep, disrupted light cycles, time zone changes, and toxic exposures.

You might have many stresses bombarding you on a regular basis, but you might not realize the toll it is taking on your body. When you're subjected to stress, particularly chronic stress, the body releases cortisol much more frequently than it should. The normal pattern for cortisol is for it to start out high in the morning, when you need the extra energy to start your day and your blood sugar is low from fasting all night.

Then, your cortisol levels normally decrease throughout the day and reach the lowest point in the evening, when you should be winding down and getting ready to go to sleep. However, under constant stress, cortisol levels are constantly high, which triggers a number of physical dysfunctions, including difficulty sleeping.

Fight or Flight: The Cortisol Response

Stressors to your body, regardless of the source, create a common response: an increased demand for the stress hormone cortisol. Your "stress response" has a number of actions. In order to accomplish them, you need a hormone like cortisol. It maintains your blood glucose during stress reactions and gives you additional glucose for use by your brain, heart, lungs, and muscles. Cortisol promotes the production of new glucose in your body at the expense of your muscles. These physical responses are important because they give you the energy to flee from danger or to fight it. However, it becomes easy to see why chronically elevated cortisol might lead to weight gain; blood sugar is increased and muscle is broken down.

Your stress response starts when the hypothalamus in your brain "sounds the alert." Your adrenal glands react by pouring out the first major stress hormone, adrenaline, which causes an increased heart rate, increased blood pressure, increased ability to clot your blood, and the release of sugar into your bloodstream. This gives you the energy to outrun your predators. The increased ability to clot your blood is helpful if you're injured during an attack.

Following the release of adrenaline, the adrenal glands discharge cortisol. Cortisol's job is to replenish the energy stores depleted by the adrenaline rush. It does this by converting a variety of food sources into storage forms like fat, increasing your activity and making you hungry. Too much cortisol enhances the storage of energy as abdominal fat. To make matters worse, the building blocks for fat production often come from the breakdown of protein in muscle. Cortisol can only increase that storage in the presence of high insulin levels. This is why the combination of insulin resistance, which causes high insulin levels, and high cortisol increases the amount of belly fat you have.

How Stress Is Related to Weight Gain

It takes a lot of energy to maintain a fight-or-flight response. Because you don't have time to create or store that energy during a crisis, your body keeps stores to draw on for emergencies. This easily accessible energy storage is in the form of simple amino acids, glucose, and fatty acids that circulate in your blood. However, your body also has more complex energy storage forms available, such as triglycerides, fat, and glycogen.

The hormone insulin stimulates the transport and storage of the simple substances into more complex forms. Insulin is an optimistic hormone that plans for your metabolic future. When you eat a large meal, insulin comes from the pancreas into the bloodstream, stimulating the transport of fatty acids into fat cells, glucose to be stored as glycogen, and amino acids to be made into proteins. The bottom line is that when insulin is present in your body, energy storage occurs, and simple building blocks of energy are stored away as more complex forms. The more stress you have, the more likely you are to keep trying to store energy for the next crisis, which contributes to weight gain.

More on Cortisol and Stress

If you used your stress response as it was designed—to outrun a predator once every few weeks—this elegant system would work well. You would store energy to be able to meet the demands of the crisis. But many misuse the stress response. People turn it off and on too often, use it for emotional tensions that are not true emergencies, or leave it on for months on end. It's an inefficient way to use energy. And those who activate the stress response too often pay a penalty for spending so much energy. They lose energy because it takes energy to keep moving nutrients into and out of the bloodstream and fuel the enzymes they need to create the complex energy storage systems. They tire more easily; they're just worn out.

Adding insult to energy, all that fat and glucose circulating in your bloodstream damages your blood vessels. And, if it is not used to outrun a predator, the extra sugar in your blood is going to eventually require insulin to store it in your cells again. This constant demand for insulin ends up contributing to insulin resistance and weight gain.

Much of the storage from high cortisol levels end up as fat around your middle. We used to think abdominal fat was just a storage depot for energy you might need later. However, we now know that fat cells are an endocrine organ (part of your hormone communication system). The fat cells communicate with your brain, and one of the main messengers is, you guessed it, cortisol.

Like many other hormone balance problems I discuss throughout this book, this scenario becomes a vicious cycle where stress and weight gain continue to feed each other. When you're stressed, your body releases cortisol, which slows down your metabolism and encourages the storage of abdominal fat. The abdominal fat, in turn, starts sending more cortisol into your bloodstream and the whole process starts again. The only way to break this cycle is to learn how to relax and reduce your cortisol demand.

Cortisol's Influence on Appetite

What we eat when we're stressed also affects our weight. If you're trying to outrun a tiger, you're probably not too hungry. The truth is about one third of us are truly not hungry during severe stress. However, two thirds of people tend to eat more than usual. This happens because the initial hormone release during the stress response stimulates adrenaline, which lowers your appetite and makes you feel jumpy and irritable, and will have your heart racing. This is a short-term response. Cortisol, the next hormone secreted, helps us to continue the stress response and start the recovery phase. Cortisol stimulates your appetite primarily for foods that are starchy, sugary, or full of fat. This helps you to replenish the stores of energy you (should have) consumed when you were dealing with your stressful situation.

Intermittent Stress

The type of stress you experience influences whether you will eat more or less during the precipitating events. For example, the typical workday for most of us features frequent intermittent stressors. Picture the example of Rhoda, who has a half-hour drive to work on an interstate highway every day. One day she sleeps too late in the morning, wakes up in a panic, hurriedly gets dressed, and hits the road as fast as she can. She feels frazzled. Then she calms down when it looks like the traffic isn't too bad, and then panics again when she sees an accident and a traffic jam ahead. She calms down when she thinks her boss isn't there and didn't see her come in late. Then she panics again when she realizes the boss did see her come in late. And so it goes on throughout the day.

Rhoda might feel like she was stressed nonstop all day. But she was actually experiencing frequent intermittent stress with frequent bursts of cortisol release and subsequent periods of lower cortisol levels. This creates a situation similar to chronically high cortisol, which promotes extra hunger and sweet cravings. Remember that part of cortisol's job is to replenish the energy used during the "alarm" phase of a fight-or-flight situation, so appetite is increased. This presents a real problem with chronic cortisol elevation.

Your Body's Personal Response to Stress

Another factor that determines how much you eat during stress is how your body responds to a particular stressor. If you put several individuals into the same stressful situation and measure their cortisol levels, you wouldn't be surprised to see that everyone has different amounts of cortisol in their systems, and the levels don't return to baseline at the same rate. These differences might be psychological, where one stressor—such as public speaking—is not too scary for one person but is absolutely terrifying for another. The difference might also be due to physiology. One person might have a liver that's slower at breaking down stress hormones or so full of other toxins that it doesn't have time to handle stress hormones as well.

A study conducted in 2001 by Epel's Group published in *Psychoneuroendocrinology* shows that women who release excess cortisol in response to stress are the most likely to overeat during these episodes. When given a number of foods to choose from during the post-stress period, they chose sweets. This effect is only seen during stress. When they are in a nonstressful situation, their cortisol levels and appetites are normal.

Eating and Emotion

Many people eat out of emotional need as much as for nutritional need. These people tend to be overweight and stress eaters. It is interesting to note that, at any given point in time, about two thirds of people are considered "restrained" eaters. This means that they're actively trying to diet or consciously trying to restrict the amount of food they consume during a meal. During stress, people who are normally restrained eaters are more likely than others to eat more.

Adrenal Fatigue

Adrenal fatigue causes a reduced production of cortisol by the adrenal gland. It can occur after stress from any source (physical, emotional, mental, or environmental) that exceeds the body's ability to adjust appropriately. When stress is chronic, the adrenal glands become fatigued and are unable to respond adequately when needed. Symptoms of adrenal fatigue include difficulty getting up in the morning, continued fatigue not relieved by sleep, craving salty foods, craving sweet foods, increased effort to do daily tasks, depression, low libido, memory less, and difficulty losing weight.

DEFINITION

Adrenal fatigue is the decrease, but not the failure, of the adrenal glands to carry out their normal function of providing the stress hormone cortisol.

Adrenal fatigue is the endpoint after long periods of unrelenting stress. Therefore, people suffering from adrenal fatigue have previously had long periods of high cortisol levels and the addition of increased fat around their middles. Because the adrenal glands and the thyroid gland are so closely tied together, their metabolism is slow and it is difficult for them to lose their belly fat.

The idea of checks and balances in the stress response is critical to its appropriate function. Too little cortisol is as bad as too much because when a stress response is insufficient, wear and tear can result. We have to keep in mind that cortisol has a number of good functions, including stabilizing the immune system and reducing inflammation. When we lack sufficient cortisol, the immune system runs wild and reacts to things that really don't pose a threat. Allergies and asthma are both considered inflammatory diseases and are classic signs of the type of problems encountered by underproduction of cortisol. Many people who suffer from these conditions notice that their symptoms worsen when they are under stress. If you are unable to lose the belly fat and notice an increase in allergies or rashes, adrenal fatigue may be your problem.

Other symptoms of adrenal fatigue include:

- Increased sensitivity to chemicals, food, and allergies
- Tendency to tremble (especially if stressed)
- Thin, dry skin
- Hypoglycemia (low blood sugar)
- Low body temperature
- Low blood pressure
- Nervousness
- Heart palpitations
- Unexplained hair loss
- Alternating constipation and diarrhea
- Indigestion

Sleep and Hormone Balance

We all know that we don't feel our best when we miss sleep. At the same time, many of us are so consistently sleep deprived that we don't remember what it is like to feel normal. America is home to the brightest, the best, and the sleepiest people in the world. A common refrain is "You snooze, you lose." In this country, it is normal for us to work at least 10 hours a day, exercise a few hours a week, and get by on five to six hours of sleep a night. We use alarm clocks, coffee, chocolate, soda, energy drinks, and many other tricks to help us "push through" the fatigue and get on with our day.

At the same time, it is becoming increasingly clear how important sleep is. Neglected sleep or poor sleep quality is a significant stressor to your body. It compromises your immune system, reduces your memory, and makes you gain weight. Just one or two nights of missed or inadequate sleep are enough to make you as insulin resistant as a type 2 diabetic! Although adequate diet and exercise can help, your physiology will never be normal without enough sleep.

Melatonin

Melatonin is an important hormone related to sleep and weight gain. To understand how it works, let's look at how our caveman ancestors lived without artificial light. As their day ended and the sun went down, the pink light of sunset came over the landscape, and they got sleepy. Sleepiness occurs because the reflected "green" light of day shuts off melatonin production. But the "rose" color of the setting sun blocks the green spectrum, causing a release of melatonin to help us get sleepy. This increase in melatonin also cools our bodies down, so we look for a warm place to snuggle and go to sleep. Part of our current hormone imbalances are due to the fact that we're surrounded by artificial light, which blocks our natural melatonin production.

The increase in melatonin, produced by the pineal gland in the brain, is important because melatonin is an initiator of sleep and a very strong antioxidant. In addition, it is produced only in the dark and if our eyes are exposed to light, we stop producing it. A study done in 2003 by Zhou showed that melatonin production naturally started declining around age 40. In some animals, melatonin has been shown to increase energy metabolism and decrease weight through the activation of brown fatty (adipose) tissue. It is not clear whether these results apply to humans yet. However, we have brown adipose tissue as well. And melatonin is closely tied to our weight in other ways.

Many of us try to cram too many things into our days and end up staying up too late and sacrificing our sleep. Also, if we have significant stress, our cortisol levels might be high, so it's difficult to settle down and nod off. We already know that decreased sleep leads to insulin resistance. So, what does this mean to our waistline?

The imbalance among insulin, cortisol, and melatonin is a recipe for disaster. Light exposure later in the evening reduces our natural melatonin production. The reduction leads to a further imbalance in insulin and cortisol. Insulin levels stay higher in the dark than they would normally, and cortisol levels fall so late they do not rise normally in the morning. This is the reversal of our normal hormone rhythms.

During the natural course of our sleep cycle, we normally wake up with high cortisol in the morning to deal with the stress of the day and with low insulin so we're hungry. However, with reversed hormone rhythms, it's easy to skip breakfast because our insulin is high and we're not hungry.

The reversal created by staying up late continues into the daylight hours when our melatonin is still too high and we need an alarm to wake up. On top of that, our cortisol is not high enough to deal with the stress during the day, so we're tired, easily overwhelmed, and unable to concentrate.

The same scenario runs again in the afternoon so that around 3 P.M., we crave carbohydrates, are inpatient with others, and have even more trouble concentrating. It's easy to see how this vicious circle continues.

Leptin is a hormone that helps us feel full and reduces appetite. Melatonin and leptin work together during the night because melatonin enhances the appetite-suppressing effects of leptin, so it's easier to stay asleep instead of waking up at night to look for food. Melatonin should enhance leptin and leptin should keep your brain from feeling hungry, so you should stay asleep and make more melatonin. Unfortunately, less sleep at night means less melatonin and less leptin, so our appetite is higher and we eat more day and night. Just losing sleep at the beginning of the night is enough to make people hungry for sugar, which leads to an increase in fat. So if you're a night owl, you might want to change your behavior!

The Least You Need to Know

- Overuse of our body's stress response results in fatigue and weight gain.
- Lack of sleep can cause weight gain and insulin resistance.
- Not enough cortisol is as bad as too much cortisol.
- Adrenal fatigue can cause fat around our middles that is difficult to remove.
- Melatonin is a hormone for sleep that requires darkness for its production; light stops its production.

Principle #5: Exercise!

In This Chapter

- The benefits of exercise
- How exercising your muscles aids your metabolism
- The importance of strength training
- How exercising your muscles makes you look trimmer
- The types of exercise that work the best

In this chapter, I discuss why exercise is Principle #5. The chapter includes information about the benefits of exercise, the relationship between your muscles and your metabolism, exercising to benefit your hormones, strength training, and interval training.

Rob's Story

Rob is a 48-year-old executive. He is the CEO of a new start-up company and works 12 hours a day, six days a week. He spends most of his time in front of his computer or at a conference table during calls overseas. When he first came to see me, he complained of lack of energy, reduced muscle mass, aching joints, and increasing belly fat. He states that he usually eats three meals and two snacks a day and works very hard to stay away from refined carbohydrates and sweets. He does confess to a "6-pack-a-day" Diet Coke habit that he's had for years. He usually sleeps about seven hours a night and doesn't have any major trouble falling asleep. He used to exercise but states that he currently doesn't have time for it, and it is difficult with achy joints.

When I spoke with Rob, we noted that his diet was actually pretty healthy except for his Diet Coke habit. We discussed the problem of caffeine increasing insulin resistance and stressing the adrenals. We also discussed the fact that artificial sweeteners and diet sodas can act like toxins in the body and create irritation and inflammation. Rob's laboratory values were normal except for some signs of inflammation, a mildly elevated fasting blood sugar, and a slightly low testosterone. He stated that he did not want to use hormone therapy, but he wanted to try and improve his overall health.

I discussed the importance of exercise with Rob. It could help him solve a number of problems without hormone therapy. Exercise, especially interval training, naturally increases testosterone and human growth hormone (HGH). It also improves insulin sensitivity. As he exercised, he would also build lean muscle mass and reduce his belly fat, which would further reduce his inflammation. After hearing the benefits of exercise, Rob decided to make time in his schedule to do an interval training program three to four times a week.

Rob also switched to seltzer water with lemon or lime and reduced his work schedule to 10-hour days, five days a week. This reduced his stress level and cortisol demand, which gave him more building blocks to produce his own testosterone. This combination of interventions had Rob looking and feeling like a new man within four months!

Rob's story shows how you can exercise your way to a healthy weight and possibly avoid hormone therapy. Exercise is the first line of defense against disease and weight problems. It is the closest thing you have to the fountain of youth. You were made to move!

How Exercise Can Affect Your Weight

The potential benefits of exercise can be difficult to imagine until you actually experience them. And if you are not a fan of exercise, getting started can be the biggest obstacle. However, it is important to make yourself do it because it dramatically enhances your hormone balance and positively affects your energy, endurance, and stamina.

Exercise plays a key role in reversing insulin resistance, increasing activity of glucagon (a fat-burning hormone), increasing testosterone and DHEA, and increasing natural HGH. It is also connected to improving cortisol balance. When people are not exercising, it is easy for these important hormones to be out of balance and create a scenario to gain weight.

In addition to hormone balance, exercise increases the amount of endorphins, natural morphinelike biochemicals that help you handle stress and improve your mood. It also raises the brain's level of serotonin, the neurotransmitter that makes you happy.

If these facts are not enough to get you moving, here are some other benefits of exercise:

- Keeps your blood sugar stable

- Controls your weight

- Controls your appetite

- Keeps your bones strong

- Prevents cancer

- Improves joint function

- Reduces the risk of stroke

- Prevents urinary incontinence

Muscle and Metabolism

According to Robb Wolf, author of *The Paleo Solution*, if you look at our initial human design, you can appreciate that, as hunters and gatherers, we needed to be active. Our genes meant for us to run, jump, fight, stalk, carry, and build. There are very few animals on this planet that don't expend significant energy finding food, avoiding danger, or looking for a mate—except for human beings. We can get by with adequate food, clothing, shelter, and safety by doing almost nothing physical. But such inactivity is very dangerous. As a matter of fact, the Centers for Disease Control list inactivity as the third leading cause of a preventable death in the United States!

Your body is an amazing machine. This fact is especially evident when you look at the skeletons from our hunter-gatherer ancestors. Their bones look like those of high-level athletes—thick and dense, which shows great strength. Even today, there are societies that still live the hunter-gatherer lifestyle with daily activities such as hunting, fishing, finding firewood and water, looking for plants, and traveling to see others. When these groups of people are tested for strength, flexibility, and aerobic ability, they do as well as highly trained athletes.

How does this happen? According to Wolf, two important factors are at work. First, the people of hunter-gatherer societies often have days of intense activity in which they walk the equivalent of 15 to 19 miles per day. Second, although some days were intense and demanding, others were relaxed and might involve almost no activity. They naturally used the important concepts of *cross-training*, which is doing more than one activity to develop fitness, and *periodization*, which is planned changes in exercise to avoid burnout.

You know strong bones are important. But some of my patients have asked me whether it really matters if their muscles are strong. It does! Muscle is one of the most metabolically active tissues in your body. It defines your metabolism. With activity, your muscle is eager to stay nourished by burning the calories you're ingesting. So the more muscle you have, the more calories you burn, whether you're at the gym, at your desk, or in your bed. If you focus on larger muscle groups such as legs, chest, back, and shoulders, you can build larger amounts of muscle in a shorter time. Also, as your larger muscles work, you increase your metabolism by continuing to burn calories even after your workout.

You need to understand two important features of muscle. First, muscle is made up of amino acids that are the building blocks for proteins and enzymes and, in times of need, glucose. Therefore, muscle provides a storage area for extra amino acids in case they are needed in times of famine or other emergency. Also, muscle has the capability to remove glucose from the blood and store it as glycogen.

When you exercise, you turn on a mechanism called *GLUT4*, which is a transport molecule on the muscle cell. The GLUT4 molecule is turned on by exercise and enables muscle cells to take in glucose without the aid of insulin. The beauty of this is that you have a decreased need for insulin and can reduce the chance of having side effects caused by high insulin levels.

DEFINITION

Cross-training is doing more than one type of activity to develop fitness.

Periodization is planned changes in exercise to avoid burnout and enhance fitness.

GLUT4 (Glucose Transporter Type 4) is a protein found in adipose tissues and striated muscle (skeletal and cardiac) that is responsible for insulin-regulated glucose translocation into the cell. In other words, GLUT4 helps glucose get into the cell.

You should be active enough so that much of your blood glucose control is handled by this mechanism. In that way, you can use the GLUT4 transport mechanisms triggered by exercise as well as insulin to help you adequately use the glucose you take in.

Unfortunately, the longer you live, the less muscle you possess, especially if you are inactive. At age 30, people who are physically inactive lose anywhere from 3 to 5 percent of their total muscle mass per decade. After the age of 50, without adequate strength training, the rate of loss doubles, translating into an average loss of 5 pounds of muscle per decade for women and 7 pounds per decade for men. This phenomenon is the biggest reason why elderly people become frail, and, because muscle dictates metabolism, is the basic cause of weight gain.

Losing muscle means losing strength, which makes any type of physical exertion more taxing and less appealing, so it breeds more inactivity. As the amount of muscle declines, a body needs less fuel from food. Therefore, even if you don't eat more, as you lose muscle, more and more of your calories will be stored as fat. On top of that, with age, your body becomes less efficient at converting the protein you eat into muscle tissue, which worsens the muscle-wasting process.

The technical term for age-related loss of muscle mass and strength is *sarcopenia*. It comes from the Greek words for "loss of flesh." This condition becomes a huge problem for elderly people who become frail to the point that they cannot get out of a chair or walk across the room without assistance. Also, this significantly increases the risk for falls and, worse yet, the fracture of bones as a result of those falls.

Frailty and sarcopenia don't develop overnight. The good news is that they can be reversed to a great degree, quite quickly, with strength training. This is true even for the elderly. Studies of nursing-home residents found that as little as two weeks of strength-building exercises, with weights or other types of resistance, can produce dramatic changes in their ability to function. If strength training can make a big difference for frail nursing-home residents, imagine how much it can do for you!

Aerobic Training

Regular aerobic exercise literally slows down the aging process. It improves the body's ability to take in and use oxygen to generate energy, otherwise known as *aerobic capacity*. Without exercise, aerobic capacity begins to deteriorate in middle age. Some researchers estimate that aerobic exercise can make your body function as though it is 12 years younger, as well as prevent major diseases and speed recovery from illness and injury. Many great activities provide aerobic exercise, including brisk walking, jogging, dancing, bicycling, skiing, tennis, soccer, and other great sports.

DEFINITION

Aerobic capacity is the maximum capacity of an individual's body to take in and utilize oxygen during exercise, which reflects the physical fitness of the individual.

The heart is the most important muscle in your body, and aerobic exercises keep it pumping at its best. To accomplish this, it's necessary to get the heart beating faster than it does during the normal course of the day. How much faster and for how long depends on what you're trying to accomplish. A difference exists between an Olympic athlete and someone who wants to try to stay fit with good hormone balance. For hormone balance and weight loss, two main objectives are key: reduce body fat or maintain it at healthy levels and keep the heart healthy.

The intensity of aerobic exercise is measured by heart rate, or the number of times the heart beats in one minute. For the best aerobic benefits, do some activity vigorously enough to make the heart beat faster than it normally does during the course of the day.

TRUSTY TIP

To calculate your maximum heart rate, use the following formula:

220 − age = max heart rate

In order to get 70 percent of your maximum heart rate, multiply your answer by 0.7. For instance, if your current age is 50, your maximum heart rate calculation looks like this:

220 − 50 (age) = 170 (max heart rate) × 0.7 = 119 (70% target heart rate)

If you want to walk aerobically without having to do math, go fast enough to breathe more than usual but still be able to talk. However, if you can still sing your favorite song, you need to go a little faster and work harder. You can monitor your heart rate by wearing a heart rate monitor, or you can check your pulse for 60 seconds and multiply it by 10.

A fit heart pumps more blood with each beat than a heart that's out of shape. Therefore, the fit heart doesn't have to work as hard at any level of activity. This means that as you become more fit, you're going to have to increase the intensity of your workout to reach your target heart rate because you're constantly improving your physical state. Monitoring your heart rate is a good way to make sure you push yourself a bit, but not too much, and increase your aerobic intensity and cardiovascular fitness at a safe pace.

Strength Training

Today, more than 40 million Americans lift weights, which is an increase of more than 60 percent from the 1970s. The most important thing about strength training is that it increases muscle mass, which is something that aerobic exercise does not do. As a matter of fact, Wayne L. Westcott, Ph.D., CSCS; Fitness Research Director at the South Shore YMCA in Quincy, Massachusetts; and the author of 20 books on exercise and fitness, states "If you only do aerobic exercise as you progress in the aging process, you will still lose enough muscle mass annually to reduce your resting metabolic rate almost as much as doing no exercise at all."

The evidence for the value of strength training has grown so much that in 2009, the American College of Sports Medicine and the American Heart Association issued new recommendations for healthy adults 65 years old and older that stress the importance of weight lifting. These groups now recommend progressing to 8 to 10 repetitions of resistance exercises for each major muscle group, including biceps, quadriceps, hamstrings, and so on. Resistance exercises should be done on two or more nonconsecutive days of the week.

Many people associate strength training with big muscles and body builders. Women are often afraid of gaining muscle and looking "bulked up." However, when women begin strength training and weight lifting, they lose body fat, gain muscle mass, and tone their body from head to toe. This is because fat takes up five times more space than muscle! So the more muscle you build, the slimmer and leaner you become.

The good news for women is that they don't have the hormone levels necessary to create the large, bulky muscles seen on men. Of course, men are free to use strength training to build those big muscles. In reality, muscles don't get stronger in the gym; they get stronger after a workout is over. When you do a strength-training workout, you slightly damage muscle fibers, which cause tiny tears in the muscle tissue. The damage to the muscle repairs itself between workouts. That is where muscle growth actually occurs. In fact, when you train with weights, you use stored body fat to fuel the repair and growth of your muscles! You can help the repair process by getting appropriate rest and adequate nutrients between workouts.

It doesn't take a tremendous amount of time and effort to reverse metabolic decline. Dr. Westcott tested a basic 10-week exercise program with 1,644 mostly sedentary people between the ages of 21 and 80. He found that at least two sessions per week in the gym—each consisting of 20 minutes of aerobics and 20 minutes of strength training—significantly improved body composition. He used two groups: one doing two workouts per week and one doing three workouts per week over 10 weeks. He found that at the end of the study, three weekly workouts produced more fat loss (4.4 pounds) compared to two weekly workouts (3.2 pounds). However, both programs added the same amount of muscle, an average of 3.1 pounds.

These statistics describe two important points. The first point is discussed by Dr. Westcott: "Other research has shown that 3 pounds of strength training increases your resting metabolic rate by 7 percent, which reverses about 14 years of the aging process." It is important to appreciate how much a small increase in lean muscle mass can improve your metabolic rate.

The second important point is that if you look at the total weight loss in either group, you see that it is not significant. The group with three weekly workouts lost 4.4 pounds of fat and gained 3.1 pounds of muscle, so the numbers on their scales only changed by 1.3 pounds. The group with two weekly workouts lost 3.2 pounds and gained 3.1 pounds of muscle, so their weight wouldn't change at all on the scale. However, you can be sure that both of these groups lost inches on their bodies because fat takes up five times the space of muscle. And their metabolic rate increased, so it will be easier for them to continue losing weight.

If you don't understand this concept and are looking for your number to go down on the scale, you are missing an important point about weight training and the beauty of building muscle. It is easy for the people in either of these groups to get frustrated by the fact that they worked out for 10 weeks and only lost 1 pound. However, they're changing their body composition, which will do great things for their overall health in the long run.

Interval Exercises

In addition to strength, other important components to fitness exist. *Power*, the ability to use strength quickly, deteriorates most rapidly with age. People have different types of muscle fibers: Type 1B, which are slow but resistant to fatigue, and Type 2A, which are fast and explosive. As you age, you naturally turn your powerful Type 2A fibers into slower Type 1B fibers, which reduces your ability to use strength quickly to accomplish tasks like jumping high or lifting heavier objects.

DEFINITION

Power is the rate at which work is done or the ability and capacity to perform work effectively.

Flexibility and range of motion are also important components of fitness. You're born as a very flexible individual. Just imagine the contortions you had to go through just to get out of the womb! As you age and spend most of your time learning and working from a seated position, you begin to tighten the muscles that help with posture and flexibility. As you continue with lack of exercise, poor diet, toxin exposure, and poor lifestyle choices, you further stiffen your muscles, which reduces your strength.

Stamina, or how your muscles work, and *endurance*, the ability of your heart and lungs to carry oxygen through your body, are also critical aspects of fitness. As you begin a fitness program, it is important to keep in mind that a balanced program enables you to optimize strength, power, flexibility, range of motion, stamina, and endurance. Interval training, which is bursts of high-intensity exercise alternated with periods of rest, is the best way to do that.

DEFINITION

Stamina is strength of physical constitution—staying power.

Endurance is the ability for someone to exert themselves for a long period of time.

Your life naturally runs in intervals. Think about how you do things if you are doing housework or yard work—you move, bend, push, walk, go upstairs, carry things from one place to another, stop for a second, and then start moving again. If you were wearing a heart rate monitor, you would see that during this time period, your heart rate and breathing are very high at some points. The same goes for children when they play many games: kickball, tag, hide and seek, jump rope, and so on. They run and stop, jump and stop, and generally move in the pattern of exertion followed by rest. Therefore, it makes sense to follow an exercise program that occurs naturally all the time, especially when you are trying to make it part of your new lifestyle.

Hundreds of studies have shown that interval training provides as good, or better, cardiovascular fitness than steady-state training exercise with no interruption, but in a fraction of the time. A fascinating study was published in 1996 in the *Medical Science of Sports Exercise Journal* by Dr. Tabata. It looked at the effects of moderate-intensity endurance training (steady-state) versus high-intensity intermittent training (intervals). This study compared a protocol of 20 seconds of high-intensity work with 10 seconds of rest repeated eight times for a total of 4 minutes of work (interval) to a protocol for 30 minutes of steady-state training. The interval group lost more fat, gained more power production, and increased aerobic capacity more than the steady-state group, and they did it in 26 minutes less per day! How did that work? The interval group, because they were training for a short period of time, trained at higher levels than could be sustained for a long period of time. This type of training is called anaerobic training, and it means that your muscles are literally working without oxygen for that time, so they work harder. The steady-state group trained at about 70 percent of their aerobic capacity, so their muscles used oxygen the whole time because they didn't have to work quite so hard.

Circuit training is the practice of performing different exercises on different muscle groups one right after another. Interestingly, we have known since the 1940s that interval weight training or circuit training is effective in building cardiovascular health, strength, and muscle. For example, you could start with leg exercises, move to arm exercises, and then to back exercises. This helps you in two ways. First, you continue moving throughout the exercises instead of resting between sets, so you keep your heart rate elevated throughout the training session. This helps to increase the amount of fat you burn and also increases cardiovascular fitness. Second, you can complete your workout in a shorter time because you are not resting between sets.

Another key part of interval training and strength training in general is compound exercises. Compound exercises use multiple muscle groups rather than focusing on one group at a time. Working out this way increases the demand on your muscles, even though you're not actually doing more work. For instance, the squat exercise actually uses more than 250 muscles! As you start to use more muscles, you use them in groups that are different from what your body is used to, which is good for developing strength. On top of that, it keeps the workout fun and interesting, which increases the chances that you'll stick with it.

The Least You Need to Know

- Regular aerobic exercise slows down the aging process.
- Muscle is one of the most metabolically active tissues in your body.
- If you lose muscle, more of the calories you consume will be stored as fat.
- It doesn't take a tremendous amount of time and effort to reverse metabolic decline.
- Interval training provides as good, or better, cardiovascular fitness than steady-state training, but in a fraction of the time.

Principle #6: Evaluate How You Eat

Chapter 9

In This Chapter

- How hormones control your appetite
- How your eating habits can affect your weight
- Why eating like a toddler is good for weight control
- The benefits of conscious eating

Your diet can have an effect on your satiety signals. Your appetite is controlled by a complex group of chemical signals among the brain, nervous system, hormones, metabolism, fat cells, and immune system. When they work well, they allow you to take in exactly as much energy as your body needs at that particular time. Many things can disrupt the signal, however, and if that happens to you, the result might be weight gain. This chapter will help you understand your satiety signals and how to rebalance them.

Alexandra's Story

Alexandra is a 24-year-old graduate student who made an appointment with me after six months of difficulty sleeping, fatigue, gas, and bloating, and a 20-pound weight gain. She is currently in a Ph.D. program at a local university and had been doing very well until, unexpectedly, she and her boyfriend separated. Prior to the breakup, her diet contained many fruits and vegetables with some breads and pastas. She also worked out two to three times a week at the university gym. After the breakup, she was very upset, had difficulty falling asleep, and woke up two or three times a night. Because of her lack of sleep, her energy declined, and she was too tired to go to the gym.

Alexandra began craving carbohydrates, and she gave herself permission to indulge in cookies and ice cream "just for a little while" because she was going through a rough time. She began to crave other carbohydrates like breads and pasta. Soon, she found that she was in the middle of eating one meal and already thinking about the next one. It seemed like she never felt full, no matter how much she ate. As the weeks continued, she felt more bloated and uncomfortable. The 20 pounds seemed to sneak on and, before she knew it, she didn't recognize herself.

When she came to see me, it was obvious that Alexandra was using food for comfort and that her body was reacting to the refined carbohydrates. Surprisingly, her laboratory values were still essentially normal. Because she was young and in good health prior to this episode, her body had not yet gotten to the point where she was sick enough to show abnormal lab values. This does not mean that she wasn't doing damage to her metabolism. The increase in weight and belly fat meant that her body was responding to an imbalance in insulin and cortisol. Her problems were being aggravated by her difficulty sleeping. Her motivation for eating was emotional rather than hunger. Therefore, it was easy for her to override her normal satiety signals. On top of that, her lack of sleep was causing a cortisol and insulin imbalance.

The first thing I did was to help Alexandra recognize that she was eating in response to emotions rather than hunger. We needed to find other outlets for her emotional turmoil. The second thing we needed to do was to help her sleep. This is an important step to help her break her cycle of craving carbohydrates.

As her sleep improved, her energy improved, and she went back to the gym, which helped her further reduce her stress. My prescription for Alexandra was to return to her diet of proteins, fruits, and vegetables and to eliminate refined carbohydrates. I also encouraged her to do a six-month trial of a gluten-free diet. Over the next six months, she lost 25 pounds and had no further bloating or abdominal discomfort. After that, she found that if she did eat any refined carbohydrates or foods containing gluten (wheat, rye, and barley), the bloating returned.

Appetite Control Mechanisms

How do you know when to eat and when to stop eating? Complex systems in your body, which use different types of chemicals to carry messages back and forth between cells, help to control your appetite. All of the cells in your body have receptors to some or all of these chemical messengers, including your fat cells.

Hormones are the messengers of your endocrine system. Certain hormones, such as leptin and ghrelin, are important for appetite control. Leptin tells your body how much fuel you have in storage and when you are full. If you lose the ability to sense leptin, appetite control is lost.

Leptin is important for both appetite and metabolism. It's made by fat cells as well as the cells lining the wall of the stomach. Leptin produced by the cells in the stomach is responsible for controlling your appetite, and when working correctly, it is effective at telling you that you are full. However, if you continue to override your natural satiety signals by eating in response to emotional issues instead of hunger, you can damage the receptor signal. You can then have a wide range of problems, including not feeling full even when you've eaten enough and craving foods like carbohydrates. In Chapter 18, we discuss how to repair those broken satiety signals.

Ghrelin tells you when you're hungry or need to take in more energy. It stimulates hunger to increase food intake and increases fat mass. It's produced by cells of the stomach lining, the pancreas, and part of the brain called the hypothalamus.

DID YOU KNOW?

Lack of sleep can cause high levels of the hormone ghrelin, which can lead to increased appetite and weight gain.

Two other hormones are central to appetite control—adiponectin and peptide YY:

- Adiponectin is a hormone that lets you know when you're full. Even though it's made in your fat cells, the less fat you have, the more adiponectin you have.

- Peptide YY is released by protein and fat intake. This hormone helps you determine when you are full. Therefore, protein and fat are more satisfying because carbohydrate intake causes very little release of this hormone. Peptide YY also works closely with leptin and makes leptin work more efficiently.

How Your Eating Habits Can Affect Your Weight

The way you eat, along with other factors—such as lack of sleep or toxin exposure—determines how much you weigh and whether you can easily take off pounds when you need to. Bad eating habits that can cause weight gain include overeating, eating foods that are not close to nature, and using food as a drug.

Overeating

If you overeat, increase your stress levels, or eat processed foods, you confuse the delicate balance among the hormones that tell you when you are hungry or full. For example, if your stress levels are high and your sleep is disturbed, the amount of ghrelin in your system will increase and make it more likely that you'll overeat and gain weight. As you gain weight, your fat cells might begin to produce more leptin. This might sound like it will lower your appetite. However, just like chronically high levels of insulin produce insulin resistance, you'll become leptin resistant if your body is exposed to large amounts of leptin over a period of time.

Eating Foods That Are Not Close to Nature

Eating foods that aren't close to nature—such as refined carbohydrates and sugars, trans fats, artificial sweeteners, and high fructose corn syrup—can quickly make people gain weight. Here's what happens:

- Refined carbohydrates and sugars create insulin and cortisol imbalance, which increases fat, especially belly fat.

- Trans fats, or partially hydrogenated oils, originally were designed by soap manufacturers. The food industry found that they significantly increased the shelf lives of food, and their use skyrocketed. Although some food manufacturers, fast-food chains, and restaurants have replaced trans fats with healthier fats, today they remain in many processed foods. Trans fats are fake and have no place in the metabolism of any living thing. They increase weight gain, reduce metabolism, and increase your risk of diabetes, heart disease, and cancer. Just say no to trans fats!

- A study from Brussels, Belgium, done in 1988 showed that artificial sweeteners like saccharine and sucralose might stimulate your taste buds and increase the production of insulin because your body thinks that something sweet is on its way and that you'll need insulin. Because the level of insulin is high, your body will start looking for more food to handle the insulin.

- High fructose corn syrup is the worst! Fructose is a natural sugar found in fruit and, because fruit also contains fiber and a number of protective nutrients, eating fructose in fruit does not create a hormone problem. However, when it's processed into high fructose corn syrup, it doesn't stimulate insulin or increase leptin, so you won't feel full. None of your appetite controls are activated when you consume foods or beverages that contain high fructose corn syrup.

Using Food as a Drug

Many people use food as a drug to feel better. Eating and drinking excessively for pleasure can lead to food addiction, which is classified by health professionals as an eating disorder. This addiction is a serious problem, and if you feel you have the problem, seek help from medical professionals who specialize in this area.

In her book *The Truth About Beauty*, Kat James discusses signs that can help you determine whether you're addicted to food:

- You need a sugar or caffeine fix to get you from lunch to dinner.
- You think about food a lot when you're not eating.
- You reward yourself with large amounts of food and then feel guilt or shame.
- You feel the urge to binge when you are upset.
- You skip meals on purpose and then gorge in one sitting.
- You get a buzz from food.
- You salivate over food advertisements.
- You prefer to eat alone, so you can eat all you want in peace.
- You obsess about your next meal even when you are full from the previous one.
- You deal with your out-of-control appetite by having nonfat frozen yogurt, large plates of vegetables, or fat-free chips.
- You worry about not getting enough food when you have to share.
- You keep eating even after you experience physical discomfort from an overly full stomach.

Food addiction is a form of self-sabotage, which is complicated because it includes your biochemistry and your emotions. On top of that, the internal voices that chide you as you have another plate of pasta, another glass of wine, or while eating your fourth pastry add to your stress level. Of course, this increases your cortisol demand and contributes to hormone imbalance.

Food addiction is a vicious cycle. For example, if you eat a sugary or starchy breakfast, you might feel a crash midmorning and reach for sweets or caffeine to jack up your sugar levels again. Then in the afternoon, the cycle repeats itself to increase your blood sugar level. The carbohydrate overload creates imbalances with insulin and cortisol. It also causes depletion of natural chemicals that allow for communication between the cells in your brain, known as neurotransmitters, which help you feel good. The feel-good neurotransmitters, dopamine and serotonin, are especially susceptible to sugar spikes, and when your diet is poor, they won't function well. When these brain messengers are affected, you're vulnerable to depression and more sugar cravings. If you can't handle the low between your fixes, you have a food addiction.

Eating Like Toddlers

Toddlers have a strong sense of when and how much they need to eat. In the first year of life, on average, a baby triples his birth weight. This is the time of fastest growth and highest need for calories per pound of body weight that people will have in their lifetime. Interestingly, as a child reaches the toddler stage, he has a naturally decreased interest in food because of slowing growth.

If you watch toddlers closely while they eat, you'll see that they focus on their food. They might pick it up with their fingers or try to use a spoon, but because self-feeding is new to them, they are present when they eat. We are innately conscious eaters. You don't see toddlers sitting in front of a television mindlessly shoving food into their mouths. Eating is an adventure for them, and they enjoy it! They inspect their food, feel it, and often wear it. You don't have to wear your food; you just need to be aware of it.

Toddlers eat small meals very often because their digestive systems are still developing, and they can't handle large amounts of food at one time. In addition, they still have intact appetite control systems. However, their consumption of empty calories should be limited so that it won't interfere with their appetites for nutritious food. Everyone should mimic this natural way of eating!

If people didn't override their toddlerlike, instinctive way of eating, they would have less trouble with weight control. The messages received as children to clean their plates, the use of food as a reward, stress eating, and not drinking adequate amounts of fluids work against the natural tendency of being present while eating.

Stress Eating

During stressful times, many people crave sweets, bread, cookies, and salty foods like potato chips or pretzels. This hunger is due to higher cortisol levels, which cause fluctuations in blood sugar and salt. Eating these types of foods creates a vicious cycle that doesn't help the stressful situation and makes the hormone imbalance worse. Above all, during stressful times, people should focus on healthy, nutritious foods that will keep their hormones balanced.

Thirst

Sometimes you might think you're hungry when the real problem is dehydration and thirst. Researchers have made interesting observations regarding hydration, thirst, and hunger. Studies show that thirst and hunger often are triggered together, so it is easy to confuse the two. Because many foods contain water, when you're eating, you might actually want water rather than the calories. To tell the difference, try drinking a glass of water if you're hungry and wait five minutes. If you're satisfied, you were thirsty.

Conscious Eating

Today's culture consists of meals on the run, fast food, energy bars, and TV dinners. The average American eats five meals a week in the car! This is a sad state of affairs when you consider the consequences: poor digestion, high cortisol levels, and distracted driving. Remember from the previous section how toddlers focus entirely on their food when they're eating. They may be squishing their peas, but they're *eating consciously.*

DEFINITION

Conscious eating is a nutrition philosophy based on the idea that listening to the body's natural hunger signals is a more effective way to reach a healthy weight than keeping track of the amounts of energy and fats in foods. It's intended to create a healthy relationship with food, mind, and body.

Many people rarely take the time to make a healthy meal, eat together, and enjoy the food that is in front of them. When you aren't paying attention to what you eat, it's easy to consume too much. In addition, much of the food you eat on the run has little nutritional value. Therefore, you remain hungry.

Conscious eating is the opposite of fast food and hurried meals. It means eating slowly, chewing well, and savoring every bite. Conscious eating and digestion start in the mouth, so it's important to chew your food slowly. In addition, while you're enjoying your food, it's important to remove as many sources of stress as possible. If your body is focusing on fight or flight, it's not focusing on the pleasure of eating and digestion.

> **THAT'S QUOTABLE**
>
> "The art of conscious eating is learning how to eat just the right amount of food to maximize every aspect of our lives. It is not a deprivation or minimal-eating diet. It is a pattern of eating that adds to our wholeness. It is a diet that requires some sensitive attention to the details of our daily activities."
>
> —Gabriel Cousens, M.D., *Conscious Eating*

As you start to slow down and listen to your body, it becomes easier to determine whether you're truly hungry or actually stressed, bored, or thirsty. In order to learn to listen to your body again, start paying close attention to the food you're craving. Often, your body is craving certain foods based on a lack of necessary nutrients.

The Least You Need to Know

- Food addiction is related to your diet, your emotional state, and your biochemistry.
- High fructose corn syrup does not activate any of your appetite control mechanisms. Therefore, it is easy to overeat when you have food or beverages with high fructose corn syrup.
- It is easy to confuse hunger and thirst. Often, when you have an increase in appetite, it is due to thirst.
- Conscious eating is an excellent way to repair damaged satiety signals.

Principle #7: Enlist the Help of Others

In This Chapter

- Why having a buddy to diet and exercise with is important
- Stopping unnecessary sacrifice
- Friends and family who try to sabotage your weight loss

People are social beings who depend on one another for support and feedback. Without support, you are more likely to abandon or fall extremely short of your goals. This chapter provides insights into why Principle #7 is so important to weight loss, exercising, and making lifestyle changes to balance your hormones.

Allison's Story

When she first came to see me, Allison, a 55-year-old housewife, was distraught over her depression, fatigue, and weight gain. Over the past 30 years, she has raised four children (ages 16 through 29) and, although she still has one child left at home, she is considering having her 85-year-old mother come to live with her. She's the responsible one in the family. She was the one who took her father to all of his doctor's appointments and cancer treatments for the three years prior to his death. During this time, her husband became distant. She doesn't feel like her marriage is doing very well at this point.

Allison has always been able to "take everything in stride." She feels frustrated that over the last year or so she hasn't had the energy or passion to do the things she needs to do for her family. She complained that she's always tired, no matter how much sleep she gets. And she has been craving carbohydrates every day at 10 A.M. and 3 P.M. If she doesn't have coffee and a candy bar at 3 P.M., she'll fall asleep.

Allison's laboratory results showed low cortisol consistent with adrenal fatigue, a high fasting blood sugar, and high cholesterol consistent with insulin resistance. Allison's adrenal glands had become fatigued through years of caring for everybody else and ignoring her own needs.

I stressed a diet of whole foods for her and told her to wean off of the refined carbohydrates and caffeine. She started some nutrients to help stabilize her adrenal glands as well (see Chapter 14). We elected to have a meeting with Allison's siblings, her husband, and her son. Upon hearing about how stressed and fatigued Allison was, her family decided to divide the care of her mother between them. In addition, her husband and son told her they would help more around the house. Allison was amazed that others were willing to help her, and she began to appreciate the beauty of asking.

The reduction in responsibilities allowed Allison to focus more on herself. She maintained a healthy diet and started taking yoga. Over the next four months, her depression and fatigue improved and she was able to lose 10 pounds. Most importantly, she began to value herself and make sure her needs were met, and she continued to help those around her.

This chapter looks at ways you can enlist the help of others to avoid the issues that Allison experienced.

How Going It Alone Affects Your Weight

Sticking to your diet, exercising, and making other lifestyle changes to optimize your hormones and lose weight can be daunting. You can find tremendous value in having a partner with whom you can face the challenge. Partnering with a buddy will help you with your diet and fitness goals; keep you on track; and lead you down the road to successful, long-term weight loss.

It is often much more difficult to remain accountable to only yourself than it is to be accountable to a friend or family member. Being accountable is key to ensuring your weight-loss efforts stay strong, sensible, and successful. Having another person to work with and listen to might keep your diet plan or exercise from becoming too extreme. If you need to explain to someone else why you can only eat cabbage on Fridays or need to be in the gym three hours a day, you're less likely to try a fad diet. Accountability works because you and your partner might be more likely to break promises to yourselves to eat better and exercise regularly, but together you'll be more likely to stick to your weight-loss routine. You don't want to let down your partner!

In a study published in 2010 in the *American Journal of Preventive Medicine*, obese women who lost 5 percent of their body weight were monitored for five years after their weight loss. Of that group, 34 percent maintained their weight loss over five years. One of the statistically significant variables to their successful weight-loss maintenance was an "increase in emotional support during that time period." According to this study, those who tried to do it alone were twice as likely to fail in their efforts to lose weight and keep the weight off.

DID YOU KNOW?

A 2007 Gallup Poll conducted for *USA Today* and *Discovery Health* of 769 Americans, ages 18 and older, who tried to lose weight shows:

- 68 percent say their circle of friends and relatives has done more to help than hinder their efforts to slim down.
- 88 percent say they've been complimented on their successes when they've been able to drop pounds.
- 57 percent say it would be helpful to them to partner with a friend or relative when trying to lose weight.

(Margin of error: 4 percent)

If you've tried to lose weight and failed, you're not alone. In fact, up to 95 percent of dieters fail within a year, and more than 70 percent of gym-goers quit in less than 90 days. Often, it seems easier to just give up or try the next fad diet again and again. This can lead to a sense of failure, increased stress levels, and further hormone imbalance with weight gain. The truth is, having a partner leads you to better weight-loss success as well as improved health, as compared to trying it on your own and running the risk of failing.

The Caretaker Role

One hindrance to making positive changes in diet and lifestyle is being trapped in a caretaker mind-set that causes you to sacrifice your own well-being. Many people were brought up to believe that they have roles to fill in their families, such as keeping the peace, protecting others from pain, maintaining a household while shielding others from the reality of bills, and other challenges. Although it is critical to work together as a family unit for the benefit of everyone, the major portion of the care should not fall on one person. This creates a great deal of stress, an increased cortisol demand, and potential weight gain.

If you're a caretaker whose motivation rests in a sense of unworthiness that requires you to provide service to others in order to prove your worth, it creates a drain on your energy. It's important to pay attention to your reasons for doing for others, especially if you're doing it to the detriment of your health. If you don't feel that you're worthy and always need to prove yourself, it will be harder for you to justify the importance of time for yourself to exercise, eat right, and recharge your batteries. As you begin to realize that you have value, you'll find it easier to ask for and accept help, which will be an important first step in helping you achieve your weight-loss goals.

Stop Unnecessary Self-Sacrifice

In her book *The Wisdom of Menopause*, Dr. Christiane Northrup discusses the fact that, in order to heal weight and digestive problems in midlife, it's necessary to pay attention to the emotional center that focuses on the balance between responsibility to ourselves and responsibility to others. This balance also affects our sense of self-esteem and is related to how we feel about our relationships, our bodies, our homes, and our lives in general.

In healthy relationships, everyone involved shares in the benefits and is able to experience improvement in life. However, many people, especially women, feel that in order to adequately care for others, they must put themselves last. A fine balance exists between nurturing others and sacrificing your own well-being in the name of caring for those around you.

When you board an airplane, the safety instructions always include, "In the unlikely event of a drop in cabin pressure, oxygen masks will fall from the ceiling. Please be sure to put on your own oxygen mask before assisting those around you." This is a great analogy for making sure that you take care of yourself first. But how many actually listen to this? To take it one step further, what if you're the pilot of the plane? What if, as the pilot of the plane, you chose to make sure all of the flight attendants and passengers had their masks on before you put yours on? What if you didn't make it back to your pilot's seat with your own oxygen mask on in time, and the plane crashed?

Did the fact that you sacrificed yourself to make sure everyone else was alright help them in the long run? The obvious answer is no. Because the pilot couldn't take care of herself first, everyone on the plane ultimately goes down. How many of you are leading a family or are responsible for others at your job? What would happen to them if you sacrificed yourself so much that your health declined or you became too stressed out to be effective?

It's important to take a close look at the balance in the things you do for yourself and for others. Everyone makes choices every day that can lead them closer to a healthy, balanced life or draw them away. You need to be honest with the motivation you have for some of your choices. Are they things you *should* do, or are they things you *choose* to do with joy? As you move away from the *shoulds* and closer to the *choices*, you'll move toward balance. In the instance of true care, motivated by choice and love, your health is enhanced, and cortisol demand is reduced.

When caring for someone gets out of balance, it's usually because the caretaker is motivated by guilt or the feeling that she should be doing it. This type of care often leads to deterioration in health and burnout. In this situation, because you didn't put yourself on the list of people who need care, your body becomes depleted. Cortisol demand goes up, you often add belly fat and increase your weight, you crave sweets, you lose sleep, and you deplete yourself of many nutrients that help run the metabolic reactions in your body.

As you continue on a path of optimal health for yourself, making yourself a priority is a critical first step. The choices you make that allow you to eat healthy, whole foods; get enough sleep at night; exercise; and do things you love to reduce your cortisol demand will ultimately help everyone around you. A beautiful side effect of optimal health is weight loss!

Get By with a Little Help from Your Friends

Often, your friends can see your strengths when you can't. As you embark on a journey to change your diet, your stress levels, your lifestyle choices, and your toxin exposures in an effort to balance your hormones, you'll need the objective eye of a support person to help you keep moving forward.

Getting the support of friends can be as important as what you're eating and how you change your lifestyle. It's paramount to your success to feel as if you're not alone in the struggle. Meeting friends for a healthy meal, exercising together, and sharing frustrations and successes are just some of the ways that enlisting help can boost your chance for success. Studies have shown again and again that people who have strong support networks do much better than those trying to make it alone with respect to weight loss, heart disease, immune system function, and brain function.

Losing weight can mean making new friends. Groups like Overeaters Anonymous and Weight Watchers are wonderful opportunities for you to meet other people who also want to lose weight. When you're among a group of like-minded people, you're sure to find them a source of motivation. Also, those with similar interests can share new ideas and information they read so that everyone can benefit.

Improving your diet and exercising with a buddy has endless benefits. You could buddy up with one person and set a date to exercise together. When you make an appointment to work out, you're far more likely to actually show up and do it! Research shows that working with a friend can help you stick to your diet, too. Friends can give you determination when temptation strikes, and they're only a phone call away. It's easier to get pumped up at first about working out or losing weight, but unless you have a friend or an accountability partner, it's hard to maintain that enthusiasm.

One of the best ways to choose the right person for the job is to identify your own problem areas. Discuss your challenges with your friend and find out what her challenges are. Then compare each other's weak spots and see whether you can complement each other. For example, if you tend to snack late at night, find a night owl whom you can call and chat with instead of raiding the refrigerator. If the vending machine at work is your downfall, a co-worker who also fights the mid-afternoon munchies will really understand and be able to help out. Ask that person to go for a walk with you during an afternoon break instead of running to the vending machine. You can also take turns bringing in healthy snacks for you both to share. With all this great camaraderie, you won't miss the vending machine!

People enjoy exercise more when they do it with a friend. You don't concentrate on the difficulty and boredom of exercising with all the fun you're having talking and socializing. Think of all the times you've run into a friend at the gym and you chatted next to each other on the treadmills, only to have your 4-mile walk fly by unnoticed. Having a workout buddy makes working out fun.

When you work with a buddy, you have someone to push you, encourage you, and motivate you. Many people find it hard to get motivated and make excuses for why they can't exercise today, or why they'll start eating healthy tomorrow. When you have a friend who's going through the same thing as you, you can encourage each other and lend support.

DID YOU KNOW?

You can encourage others around you to adopt your healthier habits. When one person slims down, those around him are more likely to lose, according to a groundbreaking study by researchers at Harvard Medical School and the University of California–San Diego. And distance doesn't matter—if you have a close friend or a sibling who lives 1 mile or 1,000 miles away, that person's weight loss or gain can have an impact on your weight.

It's also helpful to have someone to be accountable to; when someone knows what your goals are, you work harder at sticking to them because you don't want to disappoint anyone. Of course, losing weight should be about you and your health, your self-confidence, and your well-being. However, it does help knowing that at least one other person is there to hold you accountable. You're also less likely to cut corners knowing someone else is there.

Working out with a buddy is also often safer than working out alone, whether you're outside or at the gym. If walking is part of your regular routine, depending on where you live, it might be better to go in pairs or groups. It's also good if you're working in a gym or with equipment at home to have a spotter, or someone to check your form and be there if you need assistance or hurt yourself. Remember, form is important when you're doing weight lifting and resistance training. A friend can correct improper form and keep you from hurting yourself.

With a buddy at your side, you can gauge how hard you're working. Try the "breath test." Pay attention to your breathing as you exercise with your friend. If you're able to carry on a conversation or sing a song with little to no change in your regular breathing, you might not be working hard enough and need to pick up the pace a bit. On the other hand, if you can barely get a few words out because you're working so hard to breathe, you need to slow down a bit. Work toward a pace that enables you to talk in short sentences but still hold a conversation.

Another way a buddy comes in handy relates to motivation, but goes a step further to some healthy competition. If you and your friend have a little friendly competition going on—say, you bet your friend you can walk more miles, do more sit-ups, eat more servings of vegetables, or last longer on the elliptical—you can use that competitive spirit to push each other. On their own, many people won't push themselves past what they see as their own limits. However, with a little competitive encouragement, they might be amazed at what they can actually accomplish!

There are endless reasons why sharing this journey with a friend is a good idea. Everyone likes knowing that they have support and encouragement while trying to overcome unhealthy habits and making life-altering changes, both big and small. A buddy can lend the support you need while empathizing with your situation. Most people who have tried to lose weight have gone through the same experiences— setbacks, lack of motivation, lack of energy, questioning their decisions—so having someone by your side to share these experiences with makes an often difficult journey that much easier.

Friends and Family Members Who Sabotage Your Efforts

As supportive as your friends can be, a few might be sources of trouble. Many social activities revolve around food. Consider how many lunch and dinner meetings you have each week. Movies with popcorn and parties with appetizers and drinks are part of everyday life. When you start changing the way you eat, the way you relate to your friends changes, too. One of my patients talked to me about her well-meaning friends. "There were friends of mine who would pressure me to go out with them to our usual fast-food restaurants after social events or school. They thought that one meal here or there wouldn't hurt me." But the reality is that one fast-food meal can lead to another and, before you know it, you're back to your old habits.

THAT'S QUOTABLE

"Most partners, family members, and friends are very supportive. My experience is that partners want to help their loved one lose weight because they know it's important to the loved one. They want that person to be happier, to be in better health, to be more mobile, to have an opportunity to buy more appealing, attractive clothes."

—Thomas Wadden, weight-loss expert, University of Pennsylvania School of Medicine, quoted in *USA Today* on January 7, 2008

When you're trying to lose weight, you've got a lot of battles on your hands. Temptation seems to be everywhere: your pantry, your fridge, the office, and your favorite restaurant nearby. One place you're probably not expecting a challenge is among your friends. You expect your pals to be sources of empathy and encouragement, but instead, it is not uncommon to find out that not everyone in your life will support your weight-loss efforts. In fact, some people might try to make you fail.

Why would your friend try to sabotage your weight loss? Often, the reason is all too familiar: fear. Does your friend fear that the "new and improved you" will move on to things he doesn't enjoy? Perhaps a single friend fears your social life may improve, and you'll get all the hot dates. Maybe your healthier ways are making a friend feel guilty about his own less-than-perfect eating habits. Last but not least, maybe you make your friend feel better about his own weight issues when you also have one.

To keep the "old you," some pals might start trying to push food on you or suggest you remain a couch potato alongside them. It's important for you to realize that these situations can happen, recognize them, and try to understand where your friend is coming from. A key in preventing or solving this situation is communication—make it clear from the get-go that you're serious about losing weight and that you need your friends' help to make it happen.

If you recognize that someone is trying to sabotage your efforts, you have a few options. You could discuss your concerns directly with your friend or family member and ask them to support you as you take steps to improve your health. If you're uncomfortable with a direct approach, you could ask a mutual friend or another family member to speak to them. If those two avenues don't work, you may need to keep your distance from them until you reach your goals or are strong enough not to be influenced by their behavior toward you.

The Least You Need to Know

- It's important to learn to ask others for help when you need it.
- Losing weight can mean making new friends.
- Having a buddy to exercise with will make you more accountable than going at it alone.
- To prevent your friends from sabotaging your exercise, make it clear to them that you're serious about losing weight.

Putting the Principles into Action

You have looked at the seven principles of the hormone weight-loss diet. You know why you have to eat lean proteins and healthy fats. But how do you make it work? It's time to find practical ways to make eating healthy, whole foods an easy habit for you to develop and keep. This part shares some general guidelines that you can start with.

In this part, I cover how you can best arm your offense by reducing your exposure to toxins so there will be less for your liver, kidneys, and skin to handle. This part also provides information on nutrients that help support your organs of detoxification. You also find out exactly what foods you should be eating and what foods you should be avoiding.

This part also provides a quiz to find out if you have symptoms of hormone imbalance, along with tips for the best possible sleep and a wide variety of stress reduction techniques that will suit any personality or any schedule. You also learn about four important eating habits—listening to your body's cues, emotional eating, stress eating, and adequate hydration.

Finally, this part looks at how to identify the best weight loss buddy for you and how to break the ice and ask for help with a potential diet buddy.

How the Hormone Weight-Loss Diet Works

In This Chapter

- Guidelines that will make your diet a success
- Keeping a food diary
- Learning about Phases I and II
- Eating healthy foods 80 to 90 percent of the time

In previous chapters, we explored the seven principles of the hormone weight-loss diet. You know that sugar in all its forms is a dirty word, along with the word "processed." You know why you have to eat lean proteins, healthy fats, and other whole foods.

But how do you make the diet work? How do you put it all together? This chapter gives you the guidelines you should follow to make your new approach to eating a success.

Plan Your Meals in Advance

When you're trying to adopt new habits into your life, you'll be much more successful if you have a plan in place. (I've included some sample menu plans in Chapter 20 [Phase I] and Chapter 21 [Phase II].) Obviously, you don't need to follow the plans exactly—we all know that plans can change. However, if you have an idea of what you'll eat for most of your meals, it's easier to shop. And, more importantly, it limits your opportunities to give into temptation. I'm sure you know what it's like to stand in front of the cupboard or refrigerator when you're hungry and you don't know what you want to eat. That's when the less-than-optimal foods usually make their way into your mouth.

In addition to planning your meals in advance, make sure that you always have plenty of quick, easy snacks on hand wherever you are. If they're within reach, you won't give into the temptation of whatever is around. In Chapter 13, I've included lists of acceptable foods and snacks to make it easier for you to do this. Eventually, as these habits become ingrained in your daily life, you won't have to think and plan like this. But early on, failing to plan is planning to fail.

Record What You Eat

Recording what you eat in a food diary makes a big difference in your ability to lose weight. A 2001 study published in *Obesity Research* discussed the importance of dietary assessment in weight loss. Three major purposes for documenting what you eat in a food diary includes establishing a baseline of eating habits to see food patterns, monitoring for areas for improvement, and tracking progress and providing feedback. The study stated that, although it can be difficult to write everything down all the time, "when used on an ongoing basis in treatment, self-monitoring enhances weight-loss outcomes."

It's important to track your progress, especially through the first few months of the program as you begin to adjust your habits. Studies show that writing down what you eat in a food diary helps you to lose more weight. It also allows you to see patterns in your food consumption. Do you crave a specific type of food every day at the same time? Are there triggers (people, emotions, or events) that set you off and encourage poor eating habits? You also get a sense as to whether you're really hungry or not. If you want to eat something but don't want to take the time to write it down, chances are you're not really that hungry—you'll take the time if you're really hungry.

Other things that are important to track are your water and supplement intake, symptoms (digestion, allergy, emotional, rashes, headaches, mood changes, etc.) and exercise. This book has a lot of resources that can help you locate the appropriate support for you, whether it's from a friend or an online group. You can also use the Personal Action Plan form in Appendix D, which will help you document your progress.

Drink Water!

Water is critical for so many reasons. Because your body weight is made up of approximately 55 to 60 percent water, you need to make sure you get enough of it in your foods and drinks. An infant's body weight is as much as 75 percent water. However, this proportion decreases as you age. Interestingly, obesity also decreases the percentage of water in your body. Fat is a "dry" tissue with lower water content.

Water is very important for detoxification, so the lower the water content in your body, the less likely you'll be to adequately detoxify the poisons in your body. Remember, toxins are stored in your fat, and the more toxins you have, the more fat you hang on to.

In addition, studies show that increased water intake leads to more weight loss. A study done in 2008 and reported in *The Journal of the American Dietetic Association* showed that when people drank 500 milliliters of water 30 minutes prior to a meal, they ate 13 percent less food during that meal. This was unrelated to sex, age, body mass index (BMI), or daily water consumption.

Another study done in 2010 and published in *Obesity* compared two groups of dieters on reduced calorie diets for 12 weeks. In one group, the dieters consumed 500 milliliters of water prior to each main meal, and the other group did not. Over the course of 12 weeks, the group that consumed water prior to their meals lost 44 percent more weight. How easy is that? Just add the habit of drinking water prior to meals to your daily life. It's good for you in so many ways!

If you get bored with water, you can also drink hot or iced decaf herbal teas. The rule of thumb for water intake is your weight in pounds divided by 2; that is the amount of water in ounces you need. For instance, if you weigh 130 pounds, you would need approximately 65 ounces of water per day.

Eat Breakfast Every Day

Breakfast actually means "break fast"; you need to break the fast you were under as you slept during the night when your body used its readily available energy stores known as glycogen to function in the absence of regular food intake. Most nights, you deplete as much as 80 percent of those stores. If you don't eat breakfast and give your body fuel to work with, you'll quickly burn through the rest of your glycogen. Your body sees a lack of fuel as a stressor, so your cortisol level goes up, and you start to burn muscle as fuel instead. On top of that, the increase in cortisol demand contributes to overall hormone imbalance and weight gain.

Another important factor is the type of breakfast you eat. Make sure that your breakfast includes a good source of protein and healthy fats. My favorite things for breakfast include eggs, veggies, nut butters, seeds, nuts, berries, and lean meats. These will really stabilize your blood sugar much better than cereal, toast with jelly, and orange juice.

The importance of eating breakfast every morning cannot be overstated! A lot of evidence supports starting the day off with a highly nutritious meal. For example, study results published in the *Journal of Nutrition* in 2010 found that a good quality breakfast can help you to manage your appetite and reduce your risk of obesity and type 2 diabetes. Another study from 2008 reported in *Pediatrics* looked at teens over five years during Project EAT (Eating Among Teens). During the five years, they found that teens who regularly ate breakfast had a lower BMI regardless of race, sex, socio-economic status, or dietary/weight concerns. To top it off, the more often the teens ate breakfast, the lower their BMI. This happened even though the teens who ate breakfast actually consumed more calories!

THAT'S QUOTABLE

"The breakfast meal and the frequency with which it is eaten may influence appetite control, dietary intake and composition, and chronic disease risk. Breakfast skipping may lead to increased appetite, possibly leading to weight gain over time and deleterious changes in risk factors for diabetes and cardio-vascular disease. Breakfast skipping has also been linked to poorer overall diet quality. Do you need any more reasons to eat breakfast?"

—2010 Symposium Overview, Critical Reviews of Food Science Nutrition

Eat Every Three Hours

Some definite benefits are gained by eating smaller meals more frequently. Studies have shown improvement in body weight management and metabolism with smaller meals throughout the day. For example, a study in 2003 reported in the *Forum of Nutrition* states that, "increased feeding frequency leads to reduction in the total secretion of insulin and improvement in insulin resistance, and a better blood glucose control, as well as an improvement in the blood lipid profile."

The reason this approach works is that when meals are spaced in shorter intervals, there is a more consistent input of fuel. Therefore, they don't trigger an increase in cortisol demand, which would lead to fat storage and the reduction in your metabolism due to lower thyroid hormone. This also tends to keep your appetite hormones, leptin and ghrelin, better balanced. When you don't eat regular meals, the imbalance in these two hormones increases your appetite, and you're much more likely to over-eat when you finally do.

Although I am encouraging you to eat every few hours, I strongly recommend you try not to eat anything for two hours prior to going to bed. If you must have something, have a small snack with a lean protein and a healthy fat that will not affect your blood sugar or cause a spike in insulin. Your body's natural human growth hormone (HGH), which helps us build lean muscle mass and burn fat, is made during the first 90 minutes of sleep. If you had a lot of sugar prior to going to bed and have a lot of insulin in your bloodstream, you'll inhibit the production of growth hormone. In addition, the hormone ghrelin is necessary to help you sleep appropriately. So you want to have the food out of your system by the time you go to bed so you can allow ghrelin to rise.

Don't Drink Your Calories

I talked about the importance of drinking enough fluids (water and decaf herbal coffees and teas) in the beginning of this chapter. In addition to focusing on adequate water intake, you need to make sure that other beverages you drink aren't loaded with calories and sugar. Your genes have remained fairly constant over millions of years. Until very recently, the only beverage choices available were water or breast milk with occasional fruit juices available in season. Currently, a huge array of high-calorie beverages are available, and this change has shifted people's tastes and waistlines as genes and biology work every day to compensate for the liquid energies.

It's not enough just to drink adequate water; you need to make sure that you are *not* drinking other calorie-laden beverages. Since they are newer options for you (in terms of evolution), your body is not used to having such quick access to so many calories, which makes it very easy for you to gain weight.

As you work to increase your healthy habits, one of the fastest ways that you can see results is to focus on healthier beverages. If you normally drink soda, fruit juices, sports drinks, sweet tea, frozen coffee drinks, or the high-priced specialty coffee drinks, switching to seltzer water, green tea, herbal tea, and decaffeinated coffees will make a big difference for you almost immediately. Also stay away from diet sodas and diet drinks with artificial sweetener. The caffeine in them contributes to hormone imbalance because caffeine can increase insulin resistance and cortisol imbalance. Their artificial sweeteners can also act as toxins in your body.

Another major problem with drinking sweet drinks is that, without any fiber, protein, or fat, they are basically liquid sugar, which enters your bloodstream immediately. Of course, this causes a rapid rise in blood sugar, which leads to a rapid rise in insulin. The high insulin levels will do such a good job of rapidly moving the sugars from your bloodstream into your cells that your blood sugar will drop. The drop in blood sugar is a stressor on your body that causes an increase in cortisol demand, which raises your blood sugar. This see-saw effect will continue all day long with mood swings, sugar cravings, highs, and lows.

If you are currently addicted to caffeine, I recommend that you wean yourself off of it slowly. Going "cold turkey" can result in withdrawal symptoms such as headaches and agitation. Cut your caffeine dose in half every three to four days until you are almost completely off it, then stop. If you develop any withdrawal symptoms, add a little bit of caffeine back and slow your taper down (reduce your caffeine intake every five to six days instead of every three to four days).

Sugar addictions are best handled cold turkey. The first few days are difficult, but you actually lose your craving for it fairly quickly. I list the drinks that are allowed in the hormone weight-loss diet in Chapter 13.

> **TRUSTY TIP**
>
> Rather than drinking fruit juice, eat an apple, orange, or other fruit. The fiber in the fruit slows down the absorption of its sugars from the fruit into your bloodstream and does not cause the significant spike in blood sugar or insulin that fruit juice does.

Eat Healthy Foods 80 to 90 Percent of the Time

It's impossible to be perfect all the time with anything. One of the reasons that diets fail is that they're too rigid and, if you're unable to follow them perfectly, you can get frustrated and give up. After you make it through the first 30 days of Phase I of my diet (see Chapter 20), detoxify your system, and start to heal your metabolism, you can relax a little bit. Everyone has holidays, traditions, and special foods for which they need a little bit of "wiggle room." If you have been eating whole, nutritious foods 80 to 90 percent of the time, you can indulge in something special the other 10 to 20 percent of the time.

Allowing yourself room to enjoy a food that is less than healthy on occasion will reduce the chance that you'll be down on yourself because you can't be perfect. It's important to really savor that piece of birthday cake or your grandmother's famous apple strudel when you're able to indulge. Let go of any guilt! With a healthier metabolism, your body will be able to handle the occasional indulgence and you'll be able to get right back on track again.

Monitor Portion Sizes and Servings

Over the past 20 years, Americans have witnessed an increase in portion sizes as we have watched our waistlines bulge. Restaurant meals, whether at a fast-food drive-thru or a fancy sit-down dinner, have gotten larger as you equate the quality of the restaurant with getting more food for your money.

You know the words "supersize it"? This phenomenon of supersizing is a perceived value that is not limited to restaurants. The packages containing snack foods and soft drinks are getting larger and now contain multiple servings per package. With low-quality, low-cost ingredients, it's easier to make these larger packages, which appeal to Americans' sense of economic value. What's interesting is that as you look at these larger packages of food, it becomes harder to assess what a normal serving size is and even harder to only eat that amount. Following are some guidelines.

Serving Sizes

Food	Measurement Method
1 cup of salad greens	The size of a baseball
½ cup of cooked vegetables	The size of a scoop of ice cream or a light bulb
½ cup of grapes	15 grapes or the size of a light bulb
1 medium-size fruit	The size of a tennis ball
½ cup of cut-up fruit	The size of a fist
1 tablespoon of nut butter	The size of the tip of your thumb
2 tablespoons of nut butter	The size of a ping-pong ball
3 ounces of cooked meat/fish	The size of a palm or deck of cards
3 ounces of grilled fish	The size of a checkbook
1 teaspoon of butter	The size of a fingertip
2 tablespoons of salad dressing	The size of a ping-pong ball
1 ounce of nuts	The size of one handful or 2 shot glasses

Americans have a tendency to eat more when they are offered. In 2002, a study in the *American Journal of Clinical Nutrition* looked at how adults responded to meals on different days with four different portion sizes of macaroni and cheese. They discovered that the bigger the portion, the more the participants ate. As a matter of fact, they ate 30 percent more when they were offered the largest portion compared to the smallest portion. What's particularly interesting, however, is that they reported similar ratings of hunger and fullness after each meal despite the differences in how much they ate. And after the study was completed, only some of the participants even noticed that there were differences in the portion sizes served!

This phenomenon is not just limited to restaurants. Studies on portion sizes of snacks have had similar results. A study conducted in 2004 and published in *Appetite* looked at the consumption of potato chips as an afternoon snack given to men and women.

On five different occasions, men and women were given potato chips in packages that were designed to look the same except that they progressively increased in size; the largest size was more than five times as big as the smallest size. What they found was that the men and women continued to eat more at each sitting as the bag size increased. On top of that, when dinner was served several hours later, neither the men nor the women adjusted how much they ate at dinner to compensate for the difference in the amount of chips they ate. So the total calorie intake (from the snack and dinner) increased significantly for both men and women when the larger snack was eaten.

It's important to be aware of the changes in portion size and the risk of consuming more food than you need just because it's sitting in front of you. You can avoid overeating due to "portion distortion" in many ways. One of the best things you can do is learn to read food labels to determine the actual serving size and the number of servings per package. You may be surprised to find out that many bags of chips or sweetened beverages actually contain two or three servings in one package. Also, it goes back to conscious eating; instead of being distracted when you eat, be aware of where you are, what you're eating, and how you're feeling.

There are a number of ways to control your calorie intake with smaller portions:

- When in restaurants, ask for the meal to be divided in half in the kitchen before it's brought out to you. Have them plate half of the meal and put the other half into a doggie bag for you to take home.

- When at home, serve reasonable portions of food on individual plates, and keep the rest of the food off of the table instead of having it in serving dishes on the table. In addition to keeping the serving dishes off of the table, eat from smaller salad plates.

- When eating in front of the television, put a reasonable portion of food into a bowl and leave the rest of it in the kitchen. Or better yet, restrict the food you eat in front of the television.

- Because you tend to consume food more easily when you have access to it, keep healthy options like high-fiber fruits and nuts out in front.

Follow the Principles

I have laid out the seven principles to hormone balance and weight loss. As with any diet plan, true success is not related only to what you're eating. It's critical that you adjust your lifestyle as well. In addition to eating the recommended foods from

Principle #2: Eat Right (see Chapter 5), it will be important to follow the other principles as well. Action plans for each of these principles are laid out in Chapters 12 through 19. To reduce the risk of being overwhelmed, try to incorporate only one to two points from each principle into your life at once. As you become more and more comfortable with these changes, they will be easier to incorporate.

Phase I: The First Month

For the first month, focus on whole foods and eliminate two major sources of food sensitivities—dairy and grains. Removing these foods in addition to removing refined carbohydrates, sugars, trans fats/hydrogenated oils, artificial sweeteners, caffeine, and high fructose corn syrup will give your body a chance to heal. Phase I will lead to an improvement in your hormone balance, increase your metabolism, and help you lose weight. It's important for you to refrain from alcohol during this first month as well. Alcohol contains sugar, which continues your insulin imbalance. Also, because alcohol needs to be detoxified by the liver, it stresses a liver that is working diligently to remove other toxins in your body.

The first month is the detoxification phase. You remove the foods that are nutrient depleted and cause food sensitivities. Because your body doesn't need to work as hard to detoxify itself from these foods, you'll notice increased energy, mental clarity, reduced allergy symptoms, and improved digestion. Also, because grains, dairy, and toxic foods cause inflammation in your body, reducing these foods reduces your inflammation. In turn, this reduces cortisol demand, reduces fat deposition, and allows for better hormone balance. (I explained this at length in Chapter 2.)

In addition, you support your intestines as they are healing, and if, as I recommend, you use probiotics to reduce inflammation, you'll help balance out your intestinal bacteria. You have a great relationship with your intestinal bacteria and rely on them to help you appropriately digest your food. As a matter of fact, the intestinal bacteria have a huge influence on your metabolism! If you consider the bacteria within your intestines, you might be shocked to find that there are 10 times the number of bacteria inside your intestines as you have cells in your body. They actually contribute up to 3 pounds of your body weight! And they have more metabolic activity than your liver. If the bacteria are out of balance, this can create gas, bloating, poor food digestion, and nutrient depletion.

Many medications such as proton pump inhibitors used for acid indigestion and reflux cause an imbalance by reducing stomach acid. Many of the digestive enzymes used to help break down nutrients are proteins dependent on your stomach acid to activate them. If stomach acid is inadequate and the enzymes that break the proteins down are not completely activated, the proteins and nutrients are not appropriately broken down. Not only does this limit the nutrition you can get from your food, the incomplete breakdown can foster the growth of the wrong kind of bacteria in your intestines. If the wrong kind of intestinal bacteria are growing more rapidly than your helpful bacteria, it can create imbalance.

Antibiotics can also create bacterial imbalance. Since they're designed to kill bacteria, they not only kill bacteria that are causing illness, but they kill healthy bacteria in your gut as well. Even if you're vigilant about taking antibiotics only when absolutely needed, you may not realize that you currently get about 85 percent of your antibiotic exposure through your food.

Continued Success

When you're through Phase I, you've detoxified your metabolism, which is beginning to heal. Keep in mind that it took years for your hormones to become imbalanced and your metabolism to be damaged. Therefore, you won't be completely healed within 30 days. However, you can move into Phase II, which is a maintenance phase. At this point, you can eat what you ate in Phase I, and you can add back some full-fat dairy and small amounts of alcohol if you choose. Also, you can add in some gluten-free grains such as quinoa and whole-grain brown rice. If you notice that you start to gain weight again during Phase II, cut the alcohol and grains back out until your metabolism is more stabilized.

If you don't think you can survive the rest of your life on a gluten-free or dairy-free diet, re-evaluate how you feel after six months. Sometimes, after your gut has healed, you can tolerate gluten and dairy again. Of course, if you actually have celiac disease and not just gluten intolerance, you should never eat gluten.

The Least You Need to Know

- Make a diet plan in advance.
- Cut yourself some slack! Eat healthy foods 80 to 90 percent of the time.
- As with any diet plan, success is not related only to what you're eating. It's critical that you adjust your lifestyle as well.
- The first month is a time to detoxify your body by removing some of the most common sources of food sensitivity: grains and dairy.

Reduce Your Exposure to Toxins

Chapter 12

In This Chapter

- Sources of common toxins and how to reduce your exposure
- Ways to green clean your home
- Your body's detoxification organs and how to keep them working well

Living in a world that is full of toxic chemicals is dangerous and can cause you to gain weight. Fortunately, your body is well equipped to remove these dangerous toxins. However, your system can become overburdened, so the best defense is a good offense.

This chapter covers how you can best arm your offense by reducing your exposure to toxins so there will be less for your liver, kidneys, and skin to handle. It also provides information on nutrients that help support your organs during detoxification.

Reduction of Bisphenol A

Although many foods come in packaging that contains Bisphenol A (BPA), you can still reduce your exposure. The first rule is that plastic should not be heated, because it can trigger the release of chemicals. This is true even for microwave-safe containers because, although they don't disintegrate, they might still leach toxins into the food.

Depending on the brand, plastic wrap, freezer bags, and sandwich bags might leach chemicals. The National Geographic Society produces the green guide (www. TheGreenGuide.com), which provides an updated list of safe brands of freezer and sandwich bags.

Plastic storage containers have labels that identify which type of resin was used to make the container. These labels are usually on the bottom and have a triangle with a number in it. The number tells you which type of resin was used:

- Containers marked with a #2 (high-density polyethylene), #4 (low-density polyethylene), or #5 (polypropylene) are designed to be reused and do not leach chemicals.

- Bottles marked #1 (polyethylene terephthalate) are for one-time use and should not be reused; however, they are safe for the one-time use.

- Containers marked #3 (polyvinyl chloride), #6 (polystyrene), and #7 (polycarbonate) leach chemicals into the food and should be avoided. Containers marked #7 leach the most BPA. Containers marked #3 and #6 leach phthalates.

Some plastics are made from corn husks and other plants, which are a more environmentally safe, sustainable option. These are actually labeled #7 PLA, and they should be your first choice when available.

Another major place for exposure to BPA is from the lining of aluminum cans. Cans used to package many foods and sodas are lined with a resin that contains BPA. When these cans are heated to sterilize the contents, the BPA can leach from the resin into the food. Exposure to acidic or basic foods can also cause BPA to leach into the food. Therefore, foods such as tomato sauces, juices, and sodas are more likely to contain higher levels of BPA. One way to avoid this problem is to buy tomato products in glass containers or paper boxes. There is no place for soda in this diet, so you don't have to worry about replacing it.

Because our liver is fairly good at detoxifying BPA, avoiding it can cause a decrease in the total toxic load on your body. There are a number of ways that you can reduce your exposure to BPA:

- Don't microwave in plastic containers, and use glass containers. Use only containers marked with #2, #4, or #5 and don't use those marked #3, #6, or #7.

- If you can find them, #7 PLA bottles are the best to use. Drink filtered water from BPA-free and ceramic or stainless-steel bottles.

- Limit canned soups, juices, and sauces. Don't drink or eat out of Styrofoam containers.

Reduction of Phthalates

Phthalates are found in many common items used every day, including cosmetics, toothpaste, skin care products, toys, household cleaners, and many plastics. They're everywhere, and you're exposed to them regularly.

The best way to avoid phthalates is to identify less-toxic products and begin using them. Appendix B includes a list of websites and guides that can help you determine the safest products for you and your family.

Some of the more common phthalates are as follows:

- Dimethyl phthalate (DMP)

- Diethyl phthalate (DEP)

- Di (2-ethylhexyl) phthalate (DEHP)

- Monoethanolamine (MEA)

- Diethanolamine (DEA)

- Triethanomamine (TEA)

Numerous websites provide information on phthalate-free products, including cosmetics, shampoos, soaps, and household cleaning ingredients. The LessToxicGuide.ca is an excellent site, which gives information regarding all these products. Other websites are listed in Appendix B.

Some amazing things are coming to market that will help reduce your exposure to toxins. Ecovative's rice and mushroom packaging, for example, is intended to replace Styrofoam and uses an eighth of the energy required to make a similar amount of the petroleum-based stuff. And the product design consultancy The Way We See the World is working to bring edible drinking glasses made of flavored agar—similar to gelatin—to the consumer market.

You can actively reduce your exposure by making sure to read the labels on all foods and drinks so you know what you're putting in your body. Here are some guidelines to follow:

- Keep in mind that product formulations can change frequently, so keep checking labels to look for chemicals and compounds that you want to avoid.

- Make sure that you're not fooled by a label saying "natural," "green," "eco-friendly," or "botanical." Because no legal definitions for these words have been established, manufacturers of hazardous products might use these words to promote products with ingredients that aren't at all healthy.

- Third, keep in mind that "natural" is not always nontoxic. Some natural ingredients such as d-limonene, found in orange peels, are powerful solvents that can cause severe reactions in some people.

It's also important to learn to read the labels so you can make your own informed choices. In the United States and Canada, the ingredients are listed in order of quantity.

Reduction of Water Contaminants

Toxins have many ways to get into your drinking water. They can come from pesticides used on crops, leach from landfills, and come from the sewer system. Not only do you have many endocrine-disrupting chemicals in your water system, but you also have a number of pharmaceutical drugs that enter through the sewer system. Many of these chemicals are not regulated, and the water authorities don't have the technology to remove many of the toxins and medications. Therefore, you need to be responsible for your own water filtering. Several different water filters are on the market. The performance claims for a particular water purification product can be verified by reviewing the product's performance data sheet, which lists all of the contaminants the system has been certified to remove and to what percentage.

Each type of filter has pros and cons. If you are considering a filter that uses reverse osmosis or distillation, make sure that it doesn't completely demineralize the water. In nature, all water contains traces of various natural minerals such as calcium, magnesium, and potassium. These minerals are important to your overall health.

Dr. Zolton Rona, the author of *The Joy of Health*, states, "the longer one consumes distilled water, the more likely the development of mineral deficiencies and an acid state." This is because water stripped of its natural minerals is more acidic. Anytime you consume an acidic substance, your body pulls minerals from your teeth and bones to neutralize the acid. The healthiest water is produced by "selective filtration," and these products have the ability to remove contaminants and not minerals. According to WaterFilterComparisons.com, the brands of water filters that remove the most contaminants as documented by certified performance claims are Aquasauna, Culligan, and eSpring.

Don't forget about your shower! A study at Rutgers University showed that you take in as many or more chemicals showering as you do from drinking water. On top of that, when the water is hot and your pores are open, you're able to take in even more toxins such as chlorine. Also, children are more susceptible to the toxins they're exposed to during their showers and baths because they have a higher surface area to volume ratio. This means that they have more skin exposure in relation to body volume than adults do, so they can take in more toxins in relation to the body size. The three top shower filters as determined by WaterFilterComparisons.com are the Aquasauna, Jonathan Beauty Water, and Wellness Filter.

Reduce Pesticide Exposure

Pesticide exposure has been linked to a number of problems. You can reduce pesticide exposure by eating *organic* food, or if you can't afford organic, by carefully washing your fruits and vegetables.

DEFINITION

A **pesticide** is any substance or mixture of substances intended to prevent, destroy, repel, or mitigate any pest.

Organic foods are produced using environmentally sound methods that don't involve modern synthetic inputs.

A study in *Environmental Health Perspectives* by Dr. Lu and other researchers showed that when organic foods replaced most conventionally grown foods in the diets of children, in as little as five days, blood levels of key pesticides were reduced to nondetectable levels. In addition, organic foods have been found to contain more nutrients. On average, organic fruits, vegetables, and grains are 25 percent more nutritious than conventionally grown ones. Because conventional crops are bred to grow faster and larger than organic ones, the faster growth might reduce the amount of nutrients that the plant takes up from the soil. Also, because organic foods are not sprayed with chemical pesticides, they must fight harder to fend off pests, and, in the process, they produce more antioxidants.

Organic crops are produced by following some very specific criteria:

- Crops must be grown without the use of synthetic pesticides, genetic modification, irradiation, or the use of processed sewage.

- Organic farmland must be free of chemical application for at least three years.

- Livestock must eat organically grown food without any animal byproducts, must have access to pasture, and cannot be given growth hormone or antibiotics.

The following table lists the specific proportions of ingredients that must be organic in order to satisfy the label requirements.

Definition of Organic

Product Label	Proportion of Certified Organic Ingredients
100% organic	100%
Organic	95%
Made with organic ingredients	70%

Green Clean Your Home

I've already talked about the fact that many home cleaning products contain chemicals that might be harmful to you, your family, your pets, and your environment. You want to make a commitment to using fewer chemicals in the house but don't want to sacrifice cleanliness or convenience. It's never too early to start. According to the Environmental Protection Agency, the air inside your homes could have as much as 100 times the amount of pollutants as the air outside! This is due to your cleaning products, hair care products, skin care products, perfumes, and many of the other things that become volatile and get into the air.

Essential oils are derived from plants and have been around for thousands of years. They're incredibly versatile: they're antibacterial, antifungal, wonderful air fresheners, and excellent cleaners. The plants are distilled to remove the part of the plant that gives it its essence, or scent. Depending on the plant, different parts are used for the essence. For instance, rose oil comes from the petals, cinnamon oil from the bark, and lemon oil from the rind. Oils are considered essential if they carry the distinct scent of the plant from which they're derived. They're volatile and evaporate quickly at room temperature. The following table describes some excellent household uses for a number of common essential oils.

DID YOU KNOW?

Oils are highly concentrated and can irritate the skin. Therefore, you must be careful when you're handling them. When you buy essential oils, make sure that they're certified organic, therapeutic, cold-pressed oils. Store them in dark glass bottles in the refrigerator.

Oils for Cleaning and Disinfecting

Type of Oil	Household Use
Cinnamon	Antiseptic
Clove	Antiseptic, ant repellant
Geranium	Antiseptic, disinfectant, cleaner, insect repellent
Lavender	Antiseptic, antifungal, air freshener, moth repellant
Lemon and lime	Antibacterial, antiseptic, antifungal, deodorizer
Lemon grass	Antiseptic, insect repellant, cleaning agent
Oregano	Antibacterial, antiviral, antifungal, antiseptic, antiparasitic
Pine	Antibacterial, antiseptic, disinfectant, cleaner, deodorizer
Rosemary	Antiseptic, deodorizer, cleaner, dishwashing liquid, wood cleaner
Tea tree	Disinfectant, antiseptic, deodorizer
Thyme	Antiseptic, antibacterial, antimicrobial, disinfectant, cleaner
Verbena or lemon verbena	Antimicrobial, disinfectant, cleaner

It's important to keep your home smelling fresh without adding toxins. Not only are spray and plug-in air fresheners expensive, they're loaded with toxic phthalates that circulate through the air in your home. There are ways to freshen your home naturally. Potted plants are wonderful additions to your house; not only are they beautiful, scientists have found that one potted plant for every 100 square feet of your home can remove many harmful contaminants from the air. Fresh lilies and other fresh-cut flowers are visually pleasing and add the smell of flowers to your home. Another way to add a fresh natural scent is to choose an essential oil, mix it with distilled water, and put it into a spray bottle so you can spritz your carpet, linens, and other items for a fresher-smelling room.

It is possible to make your own cleaners at home with a minimal amount of energy and effort and a significant reduction in toxin exposure for you and your family. A basic shopping list includes baking soda, distilled water, organic liquid dish soap, hydrogen peroxide (35 percent food grade from a health food store), borax, lemons, spray bottles, white vinegar, and essential oils. Following are some recipes for making your own cleaners.

All-Purpose Cleaner

2 tsp. borax

4 TB. white vinegar

4 cups distilled hot water

$\frac{1}{2}$ tsp. lemon oil

2 drops pine oil

2 drops organic liquid dish soap

Mix borax into the white vinegar and hot water, stirring until it dissolves. Add oils and dish soap. Pour into a spray bottle. Do not use on Corian, granite, or marble countertops. Makes a 32-ounce solution.

Glass Cleaner

$\frac{1}{2}$ cup distilled white vinegar

2 to 3 drops lemon oil

Distilled water

Put the white vinegar and lemon oil into the 32-ounce spray bottle. Finish filling the bottle with distilled water. Shake to mix ingredients, and use. Makes a 32-ounce solution.

Shower Cleaner

1 cup baking soda

$\frac{1}{3}$ cup borax

$\frac{1}{2}$ cup liquid soap

1 cup warm water

2 TB. vinegar

4 drops pine or lemon essential oil

Mix baking soda, borax, and soap. Add warm water, mixing until the soda and borax have dissolved. Use a funnel and pour into a narrow-neck bottle. Add the vinegar and pine essential oil. Because of the combination of vinegar and baking soda, the mixture will bubble at first. Pour the mixture onto a damp cloth, clean the surface, and then rinse thoroughly. Makes a 12-ounce solution.

Toilet Bowl Cleaner

> 32 oz. All-Purpose Cleaner (see earlier recipe)
> Baking soda
> Borax

Spray the toilet bowl with the All-Purpose Cleaner. Sprinkle in a bit of baking soda or borax. Wait 5 minutes and scrub the toilet with a nylon brush.

Keep Your Detoxification Organs Healthy

Detoxification is a process by which your body transforms toxins and medications into harmless molecules that can easily be eliminated from your body. In order to be healthy and achieve weight loss, your body has to have the ability to detoxify well.

DEFINITION

Detoxification is the physiological or medicinal removal of toxic substances from a living organism.

It's important to understand how you might be exposed to chemicals, or the route of exposure. The three main pathways are: through the skin (absorption), through the lungs (inhalation), and through the mouth (ingestion). The skin is one of the most common routes of toxin exposure. Toxins can cause skin irritation, or they can be absorbed through the skin and circulate throughout the body. Inhalation through the lungs is another source of exposure. Lung tissue enables the passage of chemicals directly into the blood if they're inhaled. Some ingredients in personal care products and many ingredients in household cleaning products become airborne and create problems at home, at work, and at school. Chemicals that enter through the mouth can be ingested when they are on products you eat or drink but also with air and substances applied near the mouth, such as lipstick.

It's possible that the toxic exposure you get from your food and environment is as big a contributor to obesity as poor diet and sedentary lifestyle. Understanding the best way to keep your detoxification organs healthy and to overcome problems associated with exposure to high levels of toxic environmental chemicals will help with weight loss. The good news is that by making simple lifestyle choices and utilizing some appropriate nutrients, you can keep your detoxification organs working well and increase your body's ability to remove toxins. Common symptoms of toxin buildup in your body include headache, fatigue, muscle aches, asthma, allergies, skin disorders, and chronic infections.

Your body has four main detoxification organs: the kidney, the liver, the skin, and your gastrointestinal tract. Each of these has a different ability to break down toxins and to detoxify medications. These abilities are based on your genetic makeup but are also modified through your diet, lifestyle, and environmental exposures.

Detoxification is mainly accomplished in two phases in your liver. In Phase I, enzymes change the toxic compounds or medications into intermediate metabolites, or compounds. Phase I is the first line of defense, and if it's not functioning well, you'll have toxic buildup in your body. Many times, the inability to tolerate medication is due to a reduced ability for you to clear it from your system. In Phase II, other enzymes convert the intermediate metabolites created in Phase I into molecules that dissolve in water and can easily be removed from your body through urine or feces. This is where the kidneys and gastrointestinal tract come into play. Your skin, the fourth detoxification organ, is the body's largest absorptive organ. It lets water, minerals, medications, and toxins in and out of the body. Its main goal is to protect the body from invaders, let in water to maintain hydration, keep you cool by sweating, and remove toxins.

Supplements to Aid Detoxification

Many nutrients are needed to make the detoxification process work. If you are not well nourished and lack certain vitamins and nutrients, you might not be able to break down the toxins you're exposed to in your food and environment. The nutrients in the following table are important to help your liver's detoxification process.

Nutrients for Phase I and II Detoxification

Phase I	Phase II
Niacin	Glutathione
Magnesium	Vitamin B_6
Copper	Glycine
Zinc	Taurine
Vitamin C	Glutamine
B vitamins (B_2, B_3, B_6, and B_{12})	Folic acid
Folic acid	S-adenyosylmethionine (SAM e)

Phase I	Phase II
Bioflavonoids	Molybdenum
Alpha lipoic acid	Methionine

This is a long list of nutrients and by no means should you run to the store and buy all of these. The key nutrients listed next will make a big difference in the health of your liver.

- Herbs
- Milk thistle
- Green tea
- Vitamin C
- B vitamin complex

- N-acetylcysteine
- Alpha lipoic acid
- Bioflavonoids (citrus, pine bark, grape seed)
- Quercitin

Gastrointestinal Tract

Your gastrointestinal tract must be healthy for detoxification to work well. Can you believe that more than 400 different kinds of bacteria are in your intestines? A very fine balance exists between your gut and your immune system, and, because your gut is exposed to all the things that you eat, a chronic level of inflammation can exist. Your gastrointestinal system has a lot of influence on your metabolism, and your intestines require more energy to work than your liver does. Symptoms of an unhealthy gut include the following:

- Heartburn
- Bloating
- Nausea
- Cramping

- Abdominal pain
- Constipation or diarrhea
- Gas (flatulence or belching)
- Bad breath

Your gut might be unhealthy for several reasons. Many people have difficulties with their intestines because of poor nutrition, toxins, alcohol, antibiotics, nonsteroidal anti-inflammatory drugs like aspirin and ibuprofen, stress, low stomach acid, reduced digestive enzymes, food allergies, and travel. If the bowel remains unhealthy and full of inflammation, you can develop a condition in which the bowel allows different toxins, medications, and allergens to leak back into the bloodstream. Some doctors call this Leaky Gut Syndrome, and it can be associated with weight gain. You can gain weight because the intestine is full of inflammation that widens the junctions between the cells of the intestinal lining, allowing toxins and other allergens leaked into your bloodstream to cause inflammation throughout your body. Also, if your intestines don't have the right amount of good bacteria, you're unable to produce some vitamins, you can't adequately remove the toxins, and you can get overgrowth of more harmful bacteria and yeast.

Therefore, you need to focus on removing sources of imbalance such as poor diet, alcohol, and stress. You also need to make sure you have adequate digestive enzymes and sufficient probiotics to ensure that food is appropriately broken down and the right kinds of bacteria are present in your intestines. You can find sources for enzymes and probiotics in Appendix B.

Saunas and Steam Baths

Saunas and steam baths use your skin as a method of detoxification through sweating. As your body becomes warm and begins to sweat, you can enhance the removal of toxins. Sauna baths are an ancient tradition that has been associated with good health and healing. The tradition of the sauna goes back as far as ancient Rome with the famous Roman baths.

You have a number of options for saunas and steam rooms. Some saunas use conventional steam; others use heated rocks; and others use infrared heaters. The effectiveness of any sauna detoxification program depends on the type of heat that is used, the protocol that is used, and the type of toxins that are in the body. There are differences between a traditional dry sauna and the steam room. Although a steam room feels hotter because of the high humidity, it's actually harder for the body to sweat in the steam room than in the sauna.

Although the hot rocks sauna is still popular, it's beginning to lose ground to the more modern infrared saunas. Unlike traditional saunas that heat the body indirectly through air or steam, infrared saunas emit infrared radiating heat that's absorbed directly into the body. Sunlight is part of the wide spectrum of light frequencies, including ultraviolet and infrared light rays; infrared heat primarily warms only objects in its direct path and has a lesser effect on the temperature of the surrounding air.

In 1981, the *Journal of American Medical Association* discussed how a moderately conditioned person can sweat off 500 grams (1 pound) of fluid and consume nearly

300 calories in the sauna. Although the weight of the water loss can be regained by drinking water, the calories consumed won't be regained. Infrared saunas produce sweat that has more toxins in it. As much as 15 percent of the sweat produced in a typical infrared sauna is composed of dissolved toxins. Only 5 to 6 percent of the sweat in a traditional hot rocks sauna has toxic materials, with the remaining 94 to 95 percent composed of water.

Regardless of the method you choose, sauna treatments are good for the body and the soul. They are relaxing and are an excellent way to reduce stress. Both reducing stress and reducing the toxin load reduces your cortisol demand, helps you lose weight, and keeps your hormones balanced.

Colon Hydrotherapy

Colon hydrotherapy is a drug-free, chemical-free procedure done by a trained therapist. During this procedure, you're placed on a treatment table, a small speculum is placed in your rectum, and warm water is mixed in and out of the large intestine. The procedure takes about 45 minutes to complete, and no stress is placed on the individual during the procedure.

A number of benefits can be seen from colon hydrotherapy. Because it promotes elimination from the bowels, it's helpful for removing toxins. It's also helpful to relieve gas and bloating. And because toxins and extra wastes are removed, a number of people have seen weight loss as a result of regular colon hydrotherapy. In addition to the immediate benefits, it also helps the body to restore and repair itself over the long run. For instance, because you're removing toxins and substances that cause inflammation, your body will be better able to absorb the nutrients that you eat and maintain more healthy gut bacteria.

The Least You Need to Know

- Never heat plastic, even microwave-safe plastic.
- Toxins get into your body in three ways: through your skin, lungs, and mouth.
- Read product labels so you can make your own informed choices about what you're putting in your body.
- Make your own cleaners to reduce toxin exposure.
- Try a sauna or colon hydrotherapy to detoxify your body.

What to Eat, What to Avoid

In This Chapter

- The importance of maintaining a steady blood sugar level
- Why grains are forbidden during Phase I of the hormone weight-loss diet
- All about gluten
- Acceptable and unacceptable foods

I cannot emphasize enough how important it is to maintain a steady blood sugar level. Not only does it give the cells in your body and brain the fuel they need to function well, it also helps you avoid a large insulin response, insulin resistance, weight gain, and the blood sugar roller coaster that happens if you eat a lot of refined carbohydrates and sugars or skip meals often.

It's difficult to be on a diet for a long period of time because it's hard to remember what is allowed. The goal is to make eating to maintain a steady blood sugar so easy for you that it becomes a habit. Before you know it, you will have a much healthier lifestyle, you will lose weight, it will be easier to concentrate, you will sleep better, and your skin will look amazing!

The main goal of this book and this diet is to give you all the information you need to accomplish your hormone weight-loss goals. This chapter covers *what* to eat and *what not* to eat. In the first few weeks of the hormone weight-loss diet, refer to this chapter often to make sure you avoid the unacceptable foods and enjoy the acceptable ones.

Carbohydrates

Carbohydrates are nutrients that your body changes into glucose. The sugar is used for energy for your cells, tissues, and organs or is stored for future use. Carbohydrates are found in many food sources, such as grains and fruits.

Grains

During Phase I of the hormone weight-loss diet, you won't eat any grains—this means no wheat, rice, corn, rye, barley, or any other grains. The first 30 days are grain free because your body has a harder time processing them. They contribute to inflammation and irritation of the intestines, which can contribute to weight gain and autoimmune disease. Omitting grains for the first 30 days of the diet gives your body a chance to reduce inflammation.

After you complete the first 30 days, you can add a few whole grains. However, for the first six months of Phase II, these grains should be limited to gluten-free grains such as corn and rice. But even gluten-free grains can create inflammation. Therefore, if after adding some grains back into your diet you have a decrease in the rate of your weight loss, you might want to remain in Phase I and continue omitting grains indefinitely. You also should consider staying off grains if you have an autoimmune disease such as rheumatoid arthritis, lupus, type 1 diabetes (juvenile diabetes), Graves' disease, or Hashimoto's thyroiditis. You'll know what's right for you by how you feel.

Gluten

Gluten is a protein found in some grains such as wheat, rye, and barley. Gluten, gluten sensitivity, and *celiac disease* have recently become buzzwords. Celiac disease is a genetic intolerance to gluten, a protein found in wheat and wheat products. When I was in medical school, celiac disease was thought to be very rare (approximately 1 in 2,200 people), and the exact problem that gluten caused within the intestines was not clear. Now, it's felt to be much more common as both a genetic (celiac disease) and nongenetic (nonceliac gluten intolerance) problem.

DEFINITION

Celiac disease is a condition that damages the lining of the small intestine and prevents it from absorbing parts of food that are important for staying healthy. The damage is due to a reaction to eating gluten, which is found in wheat, barley, and rye. It also increases the risk of autoimmune disease.

According to a paper published in *Gastroenterology* in 2005, the incidence of celiac disease (caused by a genetic defect) is actually much higher, about 1 percent of the population (1 in 100, not 1 in 2,200!). And in certain Western European populations, it's even higher. It was found that celiac disease was present in 3 to 6 percent of patients with type 1 diabetes and up to 20 percent of their first-degree relatives (mom, dad, siblings, and children). They also found celiac disease in 10 to 15 percent of those with iron deficiency anemia and in 1 to 3 percent of those with osteoporosis. And for those patients who were symptomatic with intestinal symptoms, the rate of a diagnosis for celiac disease ranged from 5 to 15 percent but was as high as 50 percent in some centers!

You don't have to have the gene for celiac disease to have problems tolerating gluten. As a matter of fact, it is estimated that between 10 to 15 percent of the population has a form of gluten intolerance called nonceliac gluten intolerance. This is different from a true food allergy that results in an anaphylactic reaction. With nonceliac gluten intolerance, symptoms of food intolerances are more subtle and might take on many different forms consistent with inflammation, such as sinus congestion and stuffiness, fatigue, "brain fog" or difficulty concentrating, headaches, stomachaches, rashes, joint aches, and autoimmune diseases.

DID YOU KNOW?

You can have gluten sensitivity even if screening blood tests for celiac sprue are negative or indeterminate. Originally, screening tests for gluten sensitivity/celiac sprue consisted of blood tests against the damaging protein in gluten called gliadin. However, with heightened awareness of the possibility of gluten sensitivity in family members of diagnosed celiac disease sufferers, or in people with syndromes associated with celiac sprue, it has become clear that not all people suspected of being immunologically intolerant to gluten have positive blood tests.

So what's the problem with gluten anyway? We know that gluten is a protein found in wheat, rye, and barley. A few closely related proteins are found in spelt, kamut, and triticale. Oats do not contain gluten but are usually processed in mills that also process wheat, so they often are contaminated with gluten.

Grains actually contain a number of proteins as well. One of the protein types is called lectins. I know that it's confusing, but *lectins* are very different from the appetite hormone *leptin*. (Trust me, I didn't name all this stuff—my names would have been much clearer.) Lectins can cause a few different problems.

First, lectins are not broken down normally in the intestines as you try to digest them. Normally, you break down sugars and proteins into the basic building blocks so they can be transported out of the intestines and into the bloodstream. Lectins are able to attach to cells in the intestine and trick them into allowing the intact protein through the intestinal wall and into the bloodstream. The problem is that your body is used to seeing smaller building blocks of proteins (amino acids) instead of a large protein molecule. These intact protein molecules in the bloodstream can be mistaken for a foreign substance that needs to be "dealt with" by your immune system such as bacteria, viruses, or parasites.

The lectins, in addition to tricking the intestinal cells to transport them intact, also damage the intestinal wall so that other large proteins can sneak through as well. As your immune system mounts an attack against these proteins, it makes antibodies against them. These proteins can be similar to proteins in your body such as those found in the pancreas, thyroid, and nerve cells. So if antibodies are made against those proteins, they might also mistakenly attack important cells in your body as well. This is one mechanism by which autoimmune disease may start.

Determining If You Are Sensitive to Gluten

Blood tests can be done by your physician to determine whether you have celiac disease. However, not everyone with gluten sensitivity has a positive test showing antibodies to the damaging protein, known as *gliadin*. So if you don't test positive for antigliadin antibodies, it doesn't necessarily mean you're not sensitive to gluten.

DEFINITION

Gliadin is a glycoprotein present in wheat and several other cereals within the grass genus *Triticum*.

The best way to determine your sensitivity is to completely stop all gluten for 30 to 60 days and pay close attention to how you feel. Then you can reintroduce a food that contains gluten and see how you feel. Keep in mind you need to consume gluten only every 10 to 15 days to maintain the symptoms of gluten intolerance. Therefore, if you don't see a difference in the way you feel, make sure that you're extremely careful about reading labels so that you're not accidentally taking in gluten of which you're otherwise unaware. Gluten is contained in many different things, particularly prepared foods and sauces like some soy sauces (Tamari brand is gluten free). The best way to avoid gluten is to focus on whole foods such as meats, fruits, veggies, healthy fats, nuts, and seeds. In addition, look specifically for foods that are labeled "gluten free."

Acceptable grains include:

- Amaranth
- Brown rice
- Gluten-free oats

- Quinoa
- Sorghum

Grains and foods to avoid include:

- Bagels
- Breads
- Breakfast cereals
- Cookies
- Foods containing refined white or wheat flour and sugar

- Pastas (white flour)
- Pastries
- Processed grains

Vegetables

The two main types of vegetables are starchy and nonstarchy. It's important to know the difference because they do different things to your blood sugar levels. Starchy carbohydrates, fruits, and grains can all raise insulin levels. The *glycemic index* of each particular food item tells how much it'll raise blood glucose levels on its own. The *glycemic load* tells you how much the whole meal will raise your blood glucose level. Therefore, it's best to eat carbohydrates in combination with fats and protein, which will reduce the glycemic load and, in turn, reduce the amount of insulin the body secretes in response to the meal or snack.

DEFINITION

The **glycemic index** tells how much a food will raise blood sugar levels on its own. The **glycemic load** tells how much a whole meal will raise your blood sugar level.

The glycemic index of a food is calculated by finding the area under the curve after a number of blood glucose measurements over two hours following the ingestion of a fixed portion (usually 50 grams) of the food being studied. The area under the curve (AUC) of the test food is divided by the AUC of the standard (either glucose or white bread, giving two different definitions) and multiplied by 100. The average glycemic index value is calculated from data collected in 10 human subjects. Both the standard and test food must contain an equal amount of available carbohydrate. The result gives a relative ranking (glycemic index) for each tested food. The following table gives you the classifications for the glycemic index.

Classification	Glycemic Index Range	Examples
Low glycemic index	55 or less	Most fruits and vegetables, legumes/pulses, whole grains, nuts
Medium glycemic index	56–69	Whole-wheat products, basmati rice, sweet potato, sucrose
High glycemic index	70 and above	Baked potatoes, watermelon, white bread, most white rices, corn flakes, extruded breakfast cereals, glucose

Starchy Vegetables

Because starchy vegetables tend to have a higher glycemic index and therefore create more of an insulin response, you should eat fewer servings of these vegetables per day if you're trying to lose weight or do not have a moderate to high level of physical activity. Also, these vegetables should always be eaten in combination with fats and proteins. As always, make sure they're organic or washed well prior to eating them.

Acceptable starchy vegetables include:

- Beats
- Carrots (cooked)
- Jerusalem artichokes
- Parsnips
- Radishes
- Rutabagas

- Squash
    - Acorn squash
    - Butternut squash
    - Pumpkin
    - Spaghetti squash
    - Yellow summer squash
    - Zucchini
- Sweet potatoes
- Turnips
- Yams

If you have a significant amount of weight to lose or have diabetes, you will want to significantly restrict or eliminate these foods until your blood sugar balance stabilizes.

Nonstarchy Vegetables

The great thing about nonstarchy vegetables is that you can eat them in unlimited quantities. Eat them for every meal and snack, including breakfast. Try to eat your nonstarchy vegetables raw or lightly cooked. Make sure that they're organic or cleaned well enough to remove the pesticides. Eat at least five servings of these nonstarchy vegetables per day (feel free to eat more!).

Acceptable nonstarchy vegetables (unlimited quantities) include:

- Artichokes
- Arugula
- Asparagus
- Beet tops
- Bell peppers
- Bok choy
- Broccoli
- Brussels sprouts
- Cabbage
- Carrots (raw only)
- Cauliflower
- Celery
- Collard greens
- Cucumbers

- Eggplants
- Endives
- Green beans
- Green onions
- Kale
- Leaks
- Lettuce
- Mushrooms
- Mustard greens

- Okra
- Onions
- Peppers
- Seaweed
- Spinach
- Swiss chard
- Tomatoes
- Turnip greens
- Watercress

Fruits

Fruits are an important source of vitamins, nutrients, and antioxidants. That being said, they do affect your blood sugar and create an insulin response. However, the fructose in fruit creates a much different response in your body than high fructose corn syrup, so don't get them confused. The fiber in whole fruits slows down the absorption and reduces the insulin response more than fruit juices.

It's important to consider where you live and try to eat the fruits that are in season for your area. The recommended number of fruit servings differs based on how much weight you need to lose. (I discuss this approach in Chapter 21.)

Low glycemic index fruits include:

- Blackberries
- Blueberries
- Boysenberries

- Grapefruit
- Raspberries
- Strawberries

Medium glycemic index fruits include:

- Apples
- Apricots
- Cantaloupe
- Honeydew

- Kiwi
- Mango
- Nectarines
- Oranges

- Papayas
- Peaches
- Pears

- Pineapples (raw)
- Plums

High glycemic index fruits include:

- Bananas
- Cherries
- Dates
- Grapes

- Prunes
- Raisins
- Watermelon

Beans

Beans are packed with fiber, vitamins, minerals, and phytochemicals, which make them nutritious. Beans have significant amounts of fiber and soluble fiber, with 1 cup of cooked beans providing 9 to 13 grams of fiber. Their fiber helps you feel full for a long period of time and creates less of an insulin response in your body than many other foods.

That being said, some data shows that, like gluten, beans and legumes might create an inflammatory response in your intestines. Therefore, if you have an autoimmune disease, it might be worthwhile to eliminate beans for the first 30 days of the program and take note of how you feel when you add them back into your diet.

There is a variety of things that you can do with beans, including dips, soups, salads, and stews. The following are the most common beans we use in our foods:

- **Black beans:** Black beans are famous as the mainstay in black bean soup, a natural accompaniment to rice, and a filling in burritos and other Latin food. They're available both canned and dried in most grocery stores.

- **Black-eyed peas:** Black-eyed peas are commonly used in Southern dishes and as side dishes.

- **Garbanzo beans (chickpeas):** These acorn-shaped, yellow legumes are used in soups and as the base for hummus, a popular Middle Eastern spread.

- **Kidney beans:** Kidney beans come in a variety of colors—red, dark red, and white. The red varieties are mealy, slightly sweet, and typically used in chili dishes and soups. The white variety is milder and can become creamy when cooked well.

- **Lentils:** Lentils come in different colors and have a nutty taste. They are best in stews and salads.

- **Lima beans:** Famous for their buttery flavor, these beans are large and can be either light green or cream-colored.

- **Mung beans:** These tiny beans are commonly used in Asian dishes, often after they have sprouted. They come in several colors, such as green, black, brown, and red. The red beans (also called Adzuki beans) are used to make bean paste, a sweet paste used in Asian pastries.

- **Split peas:** This famous base for split pea soup is available in yellow or green.

Proteins

Proteins provide amino acids, which are the building blocks for muscles, some hormones, and neurotransmitters (brain chemicals). Proteins perform many other functions in your body. It's important to eat some type of protein source with each meal and snack. This helps keep blood sugar stable and slows the absorption of any carbohydrates that you eat as well. In addition, proteins send a potent satiety signal to the brain. Therefore, when you have protein in your meal, you can stay full for a longer period of time. However, you need to balance your protein intake with vegetables and fats because the liver only has the capability to process 30 to 35 percent of total calories as protein at a time.

The following are acceptable proteins:

All eggs

Acceptable meats

- Beef (organic grass fed)
- Bison
- Chicken
- Deer
- Duck
- Goose
- Lamb
- Pheasant

- Pork
- Quail
- Rabbit

- Turkey
- Veal
- White turkey

Acceptable fish

- Anchovy
- Bass
- Cod
- Fly fish
- Grouper
- Haddock
- Halibut
- Herring

- Mackerel
- Salmon
- Sole
- Tilapia
- Trout
- Tuna
- Turbot
- Walleye

TRUSTY TIP

A word about fish: salmon, herring, and mackerel are rich in omega-3 fatty acids and have been shown to reduce inflammation. Larger game fish like albacore tuna and king mackerel are at the top of the food chain and eat many other fish. Therefore, larger fish tend to concentrate mercury and should only be eaten once or twice a month. Fish known to contain less mercury are shrimp, light canned tuna, and salmon.

Acceptable shellfish

- Clams
- Crab
- Lobster
- Muscles

- Oysters
- Scallops
- Shrimp

Acceptable nuts and seeds

- Almonds
- Brazil nuts
- Cashews
- Chestnuts
- Hazelnuts
- Macadamia nuts
- Pecans
- Pine nuts
- Pistachios
- Pumpkin seeds
- Sesame seeds
- Sunflower seeds
- Walnuts

Avoid the following proteins:

- Canned tuna in oil (contains trans fats)
- Nitrate-containing products
  - Bacon
  - Canadian bacon
  - Ham
  - Hot dogs
  - Sausage
  - Soy protein isolate
- Nonorganic, nongrass-fed meats

Drinks

Your drink choices can significantly affect your diet. If you're used to consuming beverages that contain alcohol, caffeine, high fructose corn syrup, sugar, or any artificial sweeteners, you're increasing the toxin load in your body and may be sabotaging any effort to lose weight. In addition, because there is little fiber in anything you're drinking, the sugars go directly into your system and can create a significant insulin demand.

The good news is that if you have been drinking more calorie-laden, toxic beverages, you'll be able to make a big difference quickly by changing what you drink.

Acceptable drinks include:

- Cocoa Spiced Tea (made by Yogi Tea)
- Decaffeinated coffee
- Filtered water (flavored with lemon, lime, or orange slices)
- Green tea
- Herbal teas (decaffeinated)
- Sparkling waters (unsweetened)
- Steaz Diet Black Cherry Soda
- Teeccino (herbal beverage that tastes similar to coffee)
- Unsweetened coconut water (for athletes, use instead of sports drinks)
- White tea

Avoid these drinks:

- Energy drinks
- Fruit juices
- Low-fat milk
- Rice milk
- Soda/carbonated beverages
- Soy milk

Fats

It's rare that you're told by a physician to eat more fat! But that's exactly what you should do. Low-fat diets have not worked. You need fat in your diet to keep your brain and cell membranes healthy. When you eat fat with your meals and snacks, you tend to feel more satisfied for a longer period of time. The fats that are higher in omega-3 fatty acids, such as wild salmon and avocados, also help reduce inflammation in your body.

Acceptable unsaturated fats include:

- Almond oil
- Avocado oil
- Canola oil
- Grapeseed oil
- Macadamia oil
- Olive oil
- Peanut oil
- Sesame oil

Acceptable saturated fats include:

- Butter (can use in Phase I and Phase II)
- Coconut oil
- Cream (Phase II)
- Ghee (clarified butter)

Avoid these fats:

- Nonhydrogenated margarine
- Nonorganic, grain-fed animal fat (possible toxins and hormones; grain-fed animals are high in omega-6 fatty acids)
- Partially hydrogenated oils (trans fats); margarines; fast-food oils
- Refined vegetable oils (sunflower, safflower, soybean, corn)
- Vegetable shortening

Sweeteners

I have discussed how bad sugars are for you; artificial sweeteners are often worse. They're full of chemicals and toxins. A number of illnesses and side effects are connected to some of these artificial sweeteners. However, you can use a couple of natural sweeteners with this diet. Stevia is actually sweeter than sugar and comes from a shrub found in South America called *Stevia rebaudiana*. It has been used by Indians for hundreds of years and is readily available in many health food stores. Agave is another sweetener, which comes from the Mexican cactus. It has minimal impact on your insulin response and can be used in high temperatures.

Avoid these sweeteners:

- Acesulfame K (Sunette)
- Aspartame (NutraSweet)
- High fructose corn syrup
- Maple syrup
- Molasses
- Saccharine
- Sucralose (Splenda)
- Sugar

Herbs, Spices, and Condiments

It's amazing what the addition of herbs and spices can do to an otherwise boring meal! On top of that, many herbs, such as cinnamon, have health benefits. Cinnamon is known to help stabilize blood sugar and reduce insulin resistance. Turmeric and garlic are wonderful anti-inflammatory agents. Be sure to add an array of spices to food to enhance both the flavor and the healthfulness of your food.

Acceptable condiments, spices, and herbs include:

- Basil
- Bay leaves
- Cayenne pepper
- Chilies
- Chives
- Cinnamon
- Cloves
- Coriander
- Cumin
- Curry
- Dill
- Fennel
- Garlic
- Ginger
- Lavender
- Mint
- Nutmeg
- Onions
- Oregano
- Paprika
- Parsley
- Peppers
- Rosemary
- Sage
- Sea salt
- Tarragon
- Thyme
- Turmeric
- Vanilla

Avoid these condiments:

- Barbecue sauce with high fructose corn syrup
- Fat-free salad dressings with partially hydrogenated oil
- Ketchup with high fructose corn syrup

The Least You Need to Know

- Your top goal should be to maintain a steady blood sugar level.
- Between 10 to 15 percent of the population is gluten intolerant.
- To avoid an insulin response, eat only small servings of starchy vegetables.
- Eat carbohydrates in combination with fats and protein to reduce the glycemic load.
- Eat a protein source with each meal and snack to keep your blood sugar stable.

Supplements to Aid Weight Loss

In This Chapter

- The essential minerals
- How to choose a multivitamin
- How probiotics can help you lose weight
- Supplement shopping guide

Vitamins are made by living material like plants and animals. Even though they don't provide calories or directly give you energy, they ensure that thousands of reactions take place in your body to maintain a healthy metabolism, balanced hormones, and good health. Many of these reactions are linked to each other, so a deficiency of a vitamin can create a weak link in a number of chains of reactions that slow your metabolism and bring your health down along with it. This chapter gives you the information you need to supplement your daily vitamin intake and prevent deficiencies and their negative consequences.

Why Supplement?

The World Health Organization has stated that the soil in North America is barren, which means that it is 85 percent depleted in the important minerals that people need. In addition to the effects of barren soil, most of the food you buy is grown far from where you live. More important nutrients are lost as the food is processed, transported, and stored. Then people often cook it extensively, destroying even more nutrients. The following (from *Vitamins: Hype or Hope* by Dr. Pam Smith) are examples of how the nutrients in our foods can get depleted by our everyday activities relating to our food.

- Fruits and vegetables begin to lose nutritional value immediately after picking.

- Cold storage causes destruction of nutrients.

- Nutrients in some foods are not easily absorbed by your body.

- The longer you cook fruits and vegetables, the fewer nutrients remain.

Nutrient Deficiencies

Minerals and vitamins are crucial to your health. However, no government or other guidelines tell you how much of these nutrients your body requires. For example, when the recommended daily allowances (RDAs) for vitamins were developed, the purpose was to prevent people from getting diseases like scurvy and rickets, not to maximize health. And the allowances don't take into account the fact that each person needs different amounts of vitamins and nutrients depending on their unique needs.

Minerals

Minerals are solid chemical substances that have specific physical properties. They not only make up the composition of the rocks you see in nature, they are also important for your health. Four percent of your body is made up of minerals. They keep your metabolism running well, help build bones and teeth, help build hormones like thyroid, and participate in a number of reactions in your body.

There are several opinions about how many minerals are essential or required to be consumed in your diet for your metabolism to work well. Without these essential minerals, your body cannot work at full capacity and your metabolism is reduced, which leads to weight gain. The following lists essential macrominerals and trace minerals:

Macrominerals (consume more than 100 mg per day)

- Calcium
- Chlorine
- Sodium
- Potassium
- Phosphorus
- Magnesium
- Sulphur

Trace Elements or Minerals (consume very small amounts)

- Chromium
- Tin
- Zinc
- Vanadium
- Copper
- Silicon
- Manganese
- Nickel
- Iron
- Molybdenum
- Fluorine
- Iodine
- Cobalt
- Selenium

Of the 14 trace minerals listed previously, 3 or 4 may not be universally agreed on as essential, but the majority of creditable sources admit that most of them are essential. Deficiency amounts have never been determined for most trace minerals. Conclusive evidence has not been found regarding the exact daily intake amounts necessary because some of the actual requirements may be too small to measure, which is why they are called "trace."

Vitamins

Vitamins are needed in very small amounts for growth and for maintaining good health. In a study published in the *Journal of the American Medical Association* in 2002, Dr. Fletcher defined vitamin deficiency as "Suboptimal levels of a vitamin associated with abnormalities of metabolism that can be corrected by supplementation with that vitamin." In other words, if your metabolism doesn't run efficiently due to inadequate levels of vitamins, you can gain weight.

DEFINITION

A **vitamin** is an organic chemical compound that's needed for optimal function of the body. It cannot be synthesized in sufficient quantities by an organism, so it must be obtained from the diet.

Vitamins are important in many of the steps in metabolic reactions, such as burning sugars and fats for energy. Fletcher goes on to say, "Suboptimal vitamin states are associated with many chronic diseases including cardiovascular disease, cancer and osteoporosis ... Most people do not consume an optimal amount of all vitamins by diet alone ... it appears prudent for all adults to take vitamin supplements."

Another study in the *American Journal of Clinical Nutrition* published in 2010 discussed the fact that people who were on one of the popular diets like Atkins, LEARN (Lifestyle, Exercise, Attitudes, Relationships, Nutrition), and Ornish were at an increased risk for some specific vitamin deficiencies such as vitamin E, some of the B vitamins, magnesium, zinc, and iron after eight weeks. The study states, "weight loss diets that focus on macronutrient composition should attend to the overall quality of the diet including the adequacy of micronutrient (vitamin) intake." Interestingly, the Zone Diet, which doesn't omit a major food group (fat, protein, or carbohydrate), didn't show significant risk for vitamin deficiency at eight weeks. This underscores the importance of including adequate amounts of all three types of food in any nutrition plan.

Many medications deplete minerals and vitamins. Vitamins can also increase or decrease absorption of medications. Therefore, it's important to know how your medications might affect your vitamin levels and supplement accordingly if necessary. The following medications can deplete nutrients:

- Antacids can reduce folic acid absorption.

- Birth control pills deplete B vitamins.

- Estrogen replacement depletes B vitamins and increases calcium absorption.

- Methotrexate decreases beta-carotene, folic acid, and vitamin B_{12}.

- Seizure medications deplete carnitine.

- H2 blockers (for GERD) decrease vitamin D activity.

- Statin drugs deplete CoQ10.

- Diuretics deplete magnesium, potassium, sodium, and zinc.

Adapted from Vitamins: Hype or Hope *by Dr. Pamela Smith*

Safety of Supplements

It is important to make sure that supplements are pharmaceutical grade and come from high-quality sources. Although supplements are not regulated by the Food and Drug Administration (FDA), they are subject to strict labeling requirements and cannot contain any health benefit claims. Even if there is data to support a health benefit, the supplement companies cannot put that on the product labels.

THAT'S QUOTABLE

In a March 1999 Congressional hearing on dietary supplements, Rep. Dan Burton of Indiana said, "106,000 people die a year from prescription drugs, 42,000 a year from automobile accidents. It is more likely that you will be struck by lightning and die in this country than it is you will die from using a dietary supplement, with just 16 deaths reported last year."

In fact, the FDA has received only 2,621 adverse reactions since setting up a reporting system in 1993, with only 101 cases with a death reported. In some of the reported deaths, it's unlikely that the supplement was to blame, and other reports are so brief and vague it's impossible to tell.

Grades of Multivitamins

Multivitamins are available in pills, powders, and liquids, and the quantities and scope of nutrients they contain vary significantly. The choices can be confusing, but they become easier to understand after you recognize that there are basically four categories of quality for multivitamin formulations. Which one you choose depends on your own needs and budget goals. Keep in mind that the benefits come from getting these nutrients on a consistent basis.

You can consider three of the following four categories as grades of dietary supplements.

Pharmaceutical Grade

Pharmaceutical-grade supplements are available only from licensed health professionals. Some companies manufacture dietary supplements for distribution only through medical doctors and other licensed health professionals. These are the highest grade available and contain a broad range of high-quality nutrients, especially important antioxidants, and other ingredients that make it easier for a human body to use the whole formula. The manufacturers in this category make a greater investment in research related to their product formulations, in strictly controlling standards for purity, dissolution, and absorption of their products. They also focus on educating health professionals about related science. In some cases, the price tag on these multivitamins is much like some brands sold in health food stores, and in others, the health professional brands cost a little more.

Medical Grade

Medical-grade supplements are available in some practitioners' offices and higher-end health food stores and natural supermarkets. This category of multivitamins is high grade and contains well-designed, easily absorbable amounts of essential nutrients. Some brands contain a wide range of antioxidants and other beneficial ingredients not found in the low-dose variety. This category of multivitamins does not, as a rule, contain artificial flavors, preservatives, or coloring dyes.

Cosmetic or Nutritional Grade

Cosmetic- or nutritional-grade supplements are widely available in drug stores and supermarkets. The more traditional multivitamins, popularly found in these retail stores, contain very small amounts of most essential vitamins and minerals. The ingredients are often cheaper and less well absorbed. They're often not tested for purity, dissolution, or absorption. Some brands contain artificial flavors, preservatives, and coloring dyes. You can call these low-dose multivitamins, and they have the lowest price tag.

Which type of multivitamin you take depends on your personal goals. Low-dose multivitamins are designed to prevent very basic deficiencies. If you're striving for optimum health, you'll be better served by higher-quality products with a more comprehensive range of nutrients in quantities shown to enhance overall well-being.

> **DID YOU KNOW?**
>
> A study from 2005 in the *Journal of Alternative and Complementary Medicine* looked at the use of multivitamins among obese or overweight men and women over the course of 10 years. The researchers looked at 15,655 men and women from age 45 to ages 53 through 57. They noted that those who used multivitamins over the course of 10 years experienced less weight gain than individuals who do not use the supplements.

What to Look for in a Multivitamin

To support hormonal balance, weight loss, and good health, following are some of the key ingredients to look for in a multivitamin. See the "Shopping Guide" chart at the end of this chapter for quantities of each nutrient.

Vitamin A

Vitamin A and its building blocks, the *carotenoids*, support healthy eyesight, protect against heart disease and cancer, and support detoxification and thyroid function. Thyroid function is important because it enhances your metabolism and allows for weight loss. Detoxification support is also important because toxins are stored in body fat, so the fewer toxins you have, the less body fat you hang on to to protect yourself from the toxins.

Unlike carotenoids, too much vitamin A can be toxic. However, it's possible that some people don't efficiently convert carotenoids to vitamin A. A multivitamin with both vitamin A and a mixture of carotenoids is a good option. Multi-labels might list vitamin A and *beta-carotene* at the top of the ingredients list and mixed carotenoids separately, further down in the Supplement Facts panel.

DEFINITION

Carotenoids are chemicals with nutritive properties that exist in the pigment that colors plants. They are important antioxidants.

Beta-carotene is a strongly colored red-orange pigment abundant in plants and fruits and the most well-known source for pro-vitamin A.

B Vitamins

You need adequate B vitamins for efficient conversion of carbohydrates into energy and to break down fats and protein. Obviously, adequate amounts of B vitamins are critical for weight loss and helping metabolism. Collectively known as B complex, they include B_1 (thiamine), B_2 (riboflavin), B_3 (niacin or niacinamide), B_5 (pantothenic acid), B_6 (pyridoxine), B_{12} (cobalamin), and folic acid (described in more detail in the next section). The B vitamins support muscle tone in the digestive system and promote healthy eyes, skin, hair, and liver. They are also necessary for proper function of the nervous system and are good nutritional buffers against the effects of stress. B vitamins are also an important part of keeping your adrenal glands healthy. B vitamins are water-soluble, so they should be taken twice a day.

Folic Acid

Although it is a B vitamin (B_9), folic acid merits special attention because it is added to some foods, such as some cereals, and is listed separately in all multivitamins, even low-dose ones. The minimum quantity in all multivitamins is usually 400 micrograms because, when women routinely get this amount in the early stages of pregnancy, folic acid reduces the risk of their babies being born with brain and spinal defects. Because conception isn't always planned, it's advisable for all women of child-bearing age to take at least 400 micrograms of folic acid on a regular basis. For people of all ages, folic acid is associated with less risk for heart disease, depression, and Alzheimer's disease. Folic acid also helps to detoxify some hormones and environmental toxins.

Vitamin C

An antioxidant, vitamin C is especially important during times of stress, when recovering from an injury or illness, and whenever physical activity is significantly increased. Even in the best of circumstances, your body requires vitamin C for virtually every aspect of wellness, including healthy metabolism, heart function, protection against cancer, and a healthy immune system.

Low levels of vitamin C correlate with excess weight and might promote cravings for sweet or salty snacks, or beverages that are sugary or contain stimulants, such as caffeine. Because vitamin C is water-soluble, any amounts you can't absorb are excreted (extreme overdose can produce diarrhea). To use the nutrient effectively, break down your daily intake into several doses. *Bioflavonoids*, nutrients found in citrus fruits, are also antioxidants and might enhance the benefits of vitamin C. Higher-quality multivitamins often contain bioflavonoids.

DEFINITION

Bioflavonoids are ubiquitous plant compounds that are known for their antioxidant properties.

Vitamin D

As a rule, multivitamins don't contain adequate vitamin D. It was once considered to be primarily a bone-building nutrient, because it regulates calcium and phosphorus absorption. However, it also helps the pancreas release insulin, and more recent research shows that vitamin D plays a much bigger role in overall health. Endocrinologists recently have discovered that weight-loss success is more likely for those taking vitamin D. They showed that for every milliliter increase in vitamin D intake, study subjects lost nearly a quarter pound of extra weight, often in the abdominal area. Conditions linked to insufficient vitamin D include obesity and many other diseases.

> **THAT'S QUOTABLE**
>
> "Wow, where has this stuff been all these years? Vitamin D truly is the center of the universe."
>
> —Dr. Russell Chesney, professor and chairman of pediatrics at the University of Tennessee Health Science Center in Memphis

Your body makes vitamin D when your skin is exposed to sunlight without sunscreen, but few people today get enough sun to meet their vitamin D needs. In most of the United States, the sun isn't strong enough during winter months to trigger vitamin D production, and during the rest of the year, the sun poses its own risks. In food, cod liver oil, not a popular item today, is the richest source of the nutrient. Although milk and other foods are fortified with vitamin D, the amounts are relatively small. Researchers have estimated that only 4 percent of Americans over age 50 consume enough vitamin D in their diets.

Magnesium

Magnesium is needed to activate more than 300 enzymes in the body, and it helps create the structure of bones. Researchers have estimated that at least half of Americans don't get enough magnesium from their diets, which is not surprising, given that plants are the chief food source. Magnesium is important for muscle relaxation, nerve function, steroid production (sex hormones and cortisol), hormone production, energy production, and improving muscle strength and endurance. It helps to regulate levels of calcium, vitamin D, and other essential nutrients and tends to have a relaxing effect, which helps to alleviate muscle cramps and PMS symptoms, and to improve sleep. Vitamin B_6 is necessary to utilize magnesium efficiently, so it's a good idea to get at least some of the mineral in a multivitamin.

Symptoms of insufficient magnesium include chocolate cravings, PMS, constipation, depression, low energy levels, learning disabilities, excessive sensitivity to noise or pain, poor appetite or anorexia, headaches, agitation, anxiety, irritability, nausea, vomiting, abnormal heart rhythms, confusion, muscle spasm or cramps, restless leg syndrome, muscle weakness, hyperventilation, insomnia, and poor nail growth. Stress can lead to a shortfall of magnesium because it causes more of the mineral to be excreted. If you take more than your body can use, magnesium will have a laxative effect, which is easy to remedy by taking a little less.

Zinc

If your body runs low on zinc, your metabolism slows down. Another trace mineral, zinc is found in every cell and required by more than 300 enzymes in the human body for optimum function. It helps insulin to do its job and actually reduces the requirement for insulin in the body, which is critical to keep hormones balanced and reduce fat storage. It's also an antioxidant. Zinc is necessary for healthy thyroid function and metabolism, immune function, skin health, eye health, fertility, wound healing, and overall health. Although modern diets tend to be deficient in zinc, too much can create a deficiency of copper and can be toxic. Multivitamins contain copper along with zinc to maintain a balance between the two nutrients.

Calcium

In addition to being a key component of healthy bone, calcium is required for breaking up fats and energy production; normal transmission of signals through the nervous system; the transport of nutrients across cell membranes; muscle contraction, including normal heart rhythm; optimum blood clotting; and normal functioning of enzymes and hormones. To utilize the mineral effectively, your body requires adequate vitamin D and magnesium, and you're more likely to lack these other two nutrients than calcium. Excess sodium, phosphates (found in soda), alcohol, and smoking cause more calcium to be excreted and can lead to calcium depletion. Because calcium is added to many foods, including dairy products, orange juice, and some cereals, most people need less from supplements than the daily recommended total (1,000 milligrams up to age 50 and then 1,200 milligrams after). It's wise to check the calcium content of foods you eat routinely and use supplements to cover the shortfall.

Although it's important to get enough calcium, it's also possible to get too much. Excess calcium can reduce thyroid function, which might reduce your metabolism and make it more difficult to lose weight. In both men and women, some preliminary research suggests that taking too much calcium might lead to deposits of the mineral in the arteries. Too much calcium can also cause constipation.

Antioxidants

Antioxidants protect bodies from damage caused by free radicals. A free radical is an unstable molecule that reacts with oxygen in the body's cells. The molecules are unstable because they have an unpaired electron that steals a stabilizing electron from another molecule, often causing damage to the cell. Free radicals cause oxidation and are like rust on metal. They age your body and slow your metabolism.

Antioxidants work to donate stabilizing electrons to the free radicals so they can no longer damage your cells or DNA. Each antioxidant nutrient has unique qualities, and a combination offers the most protection. Beta-carotene, which gives carrots their signature color, is a precursor to vitamin A (meaning your body turns beta-carotene into vitamin A), and it's a fairly common ingredient in all types of multivitamins. However, there are other nutrients in the same family, known as carotenoids, which give plants their vivid colors and, collectively, contain a broader spectrum of antioxidants. More comprehensive multivitamin formulas contain a mixture of these, most often listed on labels as "mixed carotenoids." The key word to look for is "carotenoids," the plural being the important detail. Other antioxidants found in better-quality multivitamins but not in low-dose products include citrus bioflavonoids or bioflavonoids, lycopene, lutein, and quercetin.

Fish Oils (Omega-3s)

The omega-3 fatty acids in fish oil cool off inflammation, protect the heart, reduce physical and mental pain, decrease risk for other diseases and premature aging, and mitigate uncomfortable symptoms that often appear as hormone levels fluctuate during the course of life. Fish oil can reduce the number of hot flashes and feelings of distress, depression, and mood swings among women approaching or going through menopause, and provides relief from PMS and menstrual pain by reducing inflammation. It might also help with weight loss. A study in 2010 from the *European Journal of Clinical Nutrition* showed that women who took extra fish oils and ate more salmon lost more weight than those who didn't. Both groups were on a calorie-restricted diet. Another study from the *International Journal of Obesity* showed that the fish oil helps with the body's ability to burn fat. Those subjects that supplemented with fish oil metabolized more fat as they exercised.

Fish oil plays a key role in preventing or reversing hormonal imbalance triggered by spikes and crashes in blood sugar. The fatty acids in the oil are building blocks of cell membranes, which house receptors or doors that enable cells to receive signals and nutrients, including taking in blood glucose when it is delivered by the hormone insulin. Without healthy cell membranes, cells aren't able to function properly. In contrast to the therapeutic effect of fish oil, unhealthy fats that are prevalent in the typical Western diet can damage cell membranes, cause inflammation, and disrupt signals, which are necessary for maintaining hormonal balance and overall health.

Fish oil is the richest source of two specific omega-3 fatty acids: EPA (eicosapentaenoic acid) and DHA (docosahexaenoic acid). Although both nutrients are equally vital for good health, EPA is viewed as the key anti-inflammatory component, and DHA is vital for healthy brain function at all ages and for the development of a healthy fetus and child. EPA and DHA are classified as essential nutrients because human bodies don't make them, and diet is the only source.

Studies have found a long list of other fish oil benefits, including:

- Relief from chronic pain

- Reduced risk of diabetes

- Mood improvement and relief from depression

- Healthier skin, including relief from inflammatory skin conditions, decreased sun sensitivity, and protection against sunburn

- Prevention of osteoporosis

- Alleviation of eating disorders

- Treatment of burns

- Prevention and treatment of inflammatory bowel disease, arthritis, asthma, and muscular degeneration

When looking at different fish oil supplements, be aware that EPA and DHA, the key omega-3 fatty acids, make up approximately one third of the oil because it's found in fish. Some products are formulated to have a higher proportion of these fatty acids. Based on the research, the daily amount of a combination of EPA and DHA should be 1,000 milligrams (1 gram). To get that amount from most supplements, you need to take 3,000 milligrams (3 grams) of fish oil. When choosing a brand of fish oil, it's important to choose one of highest quality, ensuring that the oil has been properly tested for toxins and carefully handled in processing to avoid rancidity. To reap the benefits, fish oil needs to be taken on a regular basis.

Chromium

Chromium is an essential nutrient involved in the regulation of carbohydrate and fat metabolism. Chromium has been recognized for its beneficial effect on reducing blood sugar levels, burning calories, decreasing sugar cravings, reducing fat, and decreasing cortisol. Chromium appears to increase sensitivity of cells to insulin, meaning it improves cells' ability to take in blood sugar and use it as fuel for generating energy.

Given that muscle cells' refusal to accept blood sugar is a trigger of hormonal disruption as well as a key contributor to weight gain, chromium plays a key role in helping to restore and maintain balance among hormones. By stabilizing blood sugar, it might also alleviate cravings for sugary and starchy foods and help to curb an overzealous appetite.

A 1998 study in the *Journal of the American College of Nutrition* notes that "supplemental chromium has been shown to have beneficial effects without any documented side effects on people with varying degrees of glucose intolerance ranging from mild glucose intolerance to type 2 diabetes." For anyone who is diabetic, dosages of insulin or other medication might need to be adjusted when chromium is taken.

Selenium

A trace mineral (meaning it occurs in small quantities), selenium acts as an antioxidant and is required for proper thyroid function and overall wellness. It is important for the enzyme that helps convert your less active thyroid hormone, thyroxine (T4), to the much more active hormone, triiodotthyronine (T3). This conversion helps increase your metabolism and, potentially, weight loss.

Selenium content of food depends on the soil in which it's grown. Low levels are associated with higher risk for thyroid malfunction, cancer, heart disease, infection, asthma, infertility among men and women, miscarriage, depression, and rheumatoid arthritis. Getting adequate selenium might help to resolve acne and other skin conditions. It works synergistically with vitamin E, so it's a good idea to get your selenium in a multivitamin.

L-Carnitine

L-carnitine is an amino acid made from lysine, methionine, niacin, vitamin B_6, iron, and vitamin C. It's helpful for weight loss, and the usual dosage is 3,000 to 4,000 milligrams per day. The main dietary source of carnitine is red meat. Therefore, vegetarians might be low in this nutrient.

Major functions of l-carnitine include converting stored body fat into energy, reducing triglycerides, lowering total cholesterol, increasing HDL (good cholesterol), enhancing energy, and enhancing long-term memory. An animal study from 2002 showed that feeding a combination of l-carnitine and lipoic acid to rats significantly improved metabolic function and decreased oxidative stress. Fish oils have been shown to increase the efficacy of l-carnitine. If you have liver or kidney disease, you should have a discussion with your physician before starting on l-carnitine.

CoQ10

CoQ10 (*co-cue-ten*) is found in every cell and is essential for the production of energy that keeps people alive. It's used as fuel by the *mitochondria*, the energy-generating components of cells. Levels of CoQ10 start declining around age 35, paralleling the aging process and contributing to the development of heart disease and other debilitating conditions. At a minimum, low CoQ10 levels make it difficult for the human body to produce enough energy for the heart, other organs, and muscles to function well.

> **DEFINITION**
>
> **Mitochondria** are known as the powerhouses of the cell. They act like a digestive system for the cell by taking in nutrients, breaking them down, and creating energy.

Supplements are the practical way to replenish levels of the nutrient, because organ meats, which very few people eat, are the only significant food source. CoQ10 supplements have been used around the world for more than 20 years and have been found to be safe and beneficial.

Because it's so important for the energy production in your cells, having enough CoQ10 in your body ensures that you can adequately turn calories into energy. Numerous studies have found that CoQ10 significantly improves the health of people suffering from heart disease—including congestive heart failure, angina, and cardiomyopathy (a diseased heart muscle)—and aids in recovery from a heart attack. More than 1,000 heart patients have been participants in these trials.

Other research has shown that CoQ10 can help to reduce blood pressure, improve blood sugar control among diabetics, aid in breast cancer treatment, help to heal gum disease, and improve capacity to exercise. Statin drugs, used to lower cholesterol, deplete CoQ10.

Green Tea

Green tea is tea made with the leaves of *Camellia sinensis* that are specially treated and have undergone minimal oxidation during processing. It's a strong antioxidant and contains numerous catechins, the most abundant of which is epigallocatechin gallate (ECGC). Green tea also contains carotenoids; tocopherols; ascorbic acid (vitamin C); minerals such as chromium, manganese, selenium, or zinc; and certain phytochemical compounds, which produce numerous beneficial effects in the body.

A green tea extract containing polyphenols and caffeine has been shown to induce thermogenesis (creating heat by utilizing energy) and stimulate fat oxidation. It boosts the metabolic rate to 4 percent without increasing the heart rate.

A study from 2008 reported in the *American Journal of Clinical Nutrition* performed at Birmingham (UK) University showed that average fat oxidation rates were 17 percent higher after ingestion of green tea extract than after ingestion of a placebo. Similarly, the contribution of fat oxidation to total energy expenditure was also significantly higher following ingestion of green tea extract. This implies that the ingestion of green tea extract can not only increase fat oxidation during moderately intensive exercise but also improve insulin sensitivity and glucose tolerance in healthy young men.

Another study was reported in the *American Journal of Clinical Nutrition* in 2009 that looked at a combination of green tea and caffeine, which showed increased weight loss and increased fat oxidation in those that used the combination.

Probiotics

Microorganisms are tiny living organisms—such as bacteria, viruses, and yeasts—that can be seen only under a microscope. The world is full of microorganisms (including bacteria), and so are people's bodies—in and on the skin, in the gut, and in other orifices. Friendly bacteria are vital to the proper development of the immune system, protection against microorganisms that can cause disease, and to the digestion and absorption of food and nutrients. Each person's mix of bacteria varies. Interactions between a person and the microorganisms in his body, and among the microorganisms themselves, can be crucial to the person's health and well-being.

Experts have debated how to define *probiotics*. One widely used definition, developed by the World Health Organization and the Food and Agriculture Organization of the United Nations, is that probiotics are "nonpathogenic (not usually dangerous) live microorganisms, which, when administered in adequate amounts, confer a health benefit on the host." In contrast, *prebiotics* are not the actual microorganisms; they are nondigestible food ingredients that stimulate the growth of helpful bacteria already found in one's colon.

The human gastrointestinal tract contains approximately 1,012 microorganisms for every milliliter of content. Different reports state that there are between 500 and 36,000 species of bacteria living in the intestines. Essentially, the types of microorganisms you have in your intestine are usually established within the first year of your life and depend on where you live and whether or not you were breast-fed.

The delicate balance between the various types of bacteria in the intestines can be thrown off by a number of things. When antibiotics kill unfriendly bacteria so you feel better when you have an infection, they also kill the friendly bacteria in the gut. Even if you don't take antibiotics, if you're not eating organic meat, you're getting antibiotics from your food. One estimate says that people currently get 85 percent of their antibiotic exposure from meats. Unfriendly microorganisms such as disease-causing bacteria, yeasts, fungi, and parasites can also upset the balance of bacteria within the gut.

Dr. John DiBaise, in a paper published in Mayo Clinical Proceedings in 2008, stated that recent evidence suggests that the trillions of bacteria that normally reside in the human gastrointestinal tract affect nutrient acquisition and energy regulation. Therefore, the different types of bacteria inside you help determine how you absorb, store, and utilize your energy. A large body of research is beginning to demonstrate that intestinal microorganisms have an important role in regulating weight and might be partly responsible for the development of obesity in some people. It has been shown that obese people and lean people have different gut microorganisms.

Two important types of bacteria-related obesity are currently being investigated: Firmicutes and Bacteroidetes. They are the dominant bacteria in the gut. In 2005, Dr. Ley and his group published a study in the *Procedures of the National Academy of Science.* They studied mice genetically engineered to be obese and fed them the same diet as their lean siblings and mothers. When they looked at the bacteria in their intestines, they found that the obese mice had more Firmicutes bacteria, and their lean littermates had more Bacteroidetes bacteria.

In 2006, they looked at 12 obese humans on either a fat-restricted or carbohydrate-restricted diet for a year. Before diet therapy, obese patients had more Firmicutes and less Bacteroidetes than lean participants used as controls. After weight loss, the relative proportion of Bacteroidetes increased and Firmicutes decreased. The shift in percentage to the "leaner" Bacteroidetes correlated with the percentage of weight lost and not with the dietary changes in calorie content.

You need to make sure that you're working to keep your intestinal bacteria in balance. You can do so by consuming a diet of whole, organic foods and limiting sugars and toxins. You might be able to increase your levels of healthy intestinal bacteria by consuming some specific foods as well. Examples of foods containing probiotics are yogurt, fermented and unfermented milk, miso, tempeh, and some juices and soy beverages.

In probiotic foods and supplements, the bacteria might have been present originally or added during preparation. I recommend probiotic supplements that are pharmaceutical grade and contain at least a billion cfu (colony forming units) of bacteria per dose.

Timing of Supplementation

As a rule, supplements are used more effectively if taken with food, and any ingredients that help your body to generate energy should be taken early in the day. For example:

- If your multivitamin consists of one pill, take it with breakfast, and if a daily serving is more than one pill, take half with breakfast and the rest with lunch. It's best not to take multivitamins later in the day because B vitamins improve energy, and there's a chance that they might keep you up if taken late in the day.

- Take CoQ10 in the morning, because it enhances energy production. To absorb it well, take CoQ10 with some food that contains a little fat.

- Take your extra vitamin D at the same time as your multivitamin so it's more convenient.

- If your daily serving of fish oil consists of several capsules, split these among breakfast, lunch, and dinner. Some people find that taking too much fish oil at once makes them burp.

- Extra vitamin C and calcium won't interfere with sleep and can be taken anytime, preferably with food.

- For better sleep, take 400 milligrams of magnesium glycinate or 600 milligrams of magnesium oxide in the evening.

Supplement Shopping Guide

These are some key ingredients to look for in a good quality multivitamin. The amounts of each nutrient are a rough guide.

Supplement Guide

Nutrient	Approximate Quantity per Serving Size
Vitamin A, beta-carotene, and other carotenoids	5,000 IU or less of vitamin A; up to 15,000 IU of mixed
B vitamins	50–100 mg of B_1 (thiamine), B_2 (riboflavin), B_3 (niacin or niacinamide), B_5 (pantothenic acid), and B_6 (pyridoxine); up to 1,000 mcg of B_{12} (cobalamin)
Folic acid	800 mcg
Vitamin C	1,000–2,000 mg daily, divided into several doses; up to 5,000 mg during times of stress, from a multi and additional vitamin C supplements
Vitamin D	1,000–2,000 IU daily of the D_3 form (cholecalciferol), from a multi and additional vitamin D supplements
Vitamin E	200–400 IU of a combination of vitamin E and mixed tocopherols
Calcium	500–1,000 mg (depending on age and menopausal status)
Magnesium	At least 250 mg
Chromium	At least 200 mcg
Selenium	200 mcg
Zinc	20 to 40 mg
Iodine	150 to 200 mcg

In Addition to a Multivitamin

Some products provide daily servings of a variety of vitamins, minerals, and fish oil in a packet-a-day format, rather than a bottle of pills, and the packets might contain everything you need. Otherwise, you need to take some individual nutrients separately in addition to a multivitamin, including:

- **Extra vitamin C:** Add to your multivitamin daily if needed and take extra C in times of stress.

- **Extra vitamin D:** Multivitamins don't usually contain adequate amounts, so add enough to get 1,000 to 2,000 IU total daily.

- **Extra calcium:** Aim for 1,000 milligrams daily up to age 50 and 1,200 milligrams after that, from a combination of food and supplements. Supplements should only make up for any shortfall from food, and you might not need more than the amount in a multivitamin.

- **Extra magnesium:** Aim to get 400 milligrams twice daily of the glycinate form or 600 milligrams twice daily of the oxide form, from a combination of a multi and additional magnesium supplements. If diarrhea occurs, reduce the amount.

- **Fish oil:** Take 3,000 milligrams (3 grams) and 5,000 milligrams (5 grams) when PMS symptoms begin.

- **CoQ10:** After age 35, take 50 milligrams or, if you're overweight or have high blood pressure, fatigue, diabetes, or any form of heart disease or other illness, take 100 to 200 milligrams.

- **Flaxseed oil (optional):** Take 1 to 2 tablespoons daily or the equivalent in capsule form.

The Least You Need to Know

- It's important to buy the highest-quality supplements you can afford, especially for fish oils.

- Essential minerals are required for your metabolism to work well. They must be consumed in your diet or taken as a supplement. Without these essential minerals, your body cannot work at full capacity.

- Two important types of bacteria in the gut, Firmicutes and Bacteroidetes, are being investigated for their potential role in obesity.
- Each antioxidant nutrient has unique qualities, and a combination offers the most protection.

Find Out Whether Your Hormones Are in Balance

In This Chapter

- Testing hormone levels
- A quiz to identify possible hormone imbalance
- Other tests that reveal possible hormone-related problems

This book is about the role hormones play in your body and how they affect your metabolism, mood, weight, energy level, sleep, and even your susceptibility to disease. This chapter gives you the information you need to determine what your hormone levels are and whether they are in balance.

Hormone Testing

Take the following quiz to see whether you have hormone imbalances. If the scores and the interpretation indicate you might have a problem, it might be worthwhile to have your hormone levels checked to see exactly which ones are too high or too low. (I discussed the various types of hormone tests, including blood, urine, and saliva, in Chapter 6.)

I encourage you to speak to your physician regarding the evaluation of your hormone levels. If your physician is unable to help you with these types of tests, contact one of the laboratories listed in Appendix B, and they'll be able to help you.

Hormone Balance Quiz

The following quiz has 10 sections, each of which represents a different hormone imbalance that might affect your ability to lose weight. Answer each question by checking Always, Sometimes, or Never as it pertains to you. At the end of the quiz, I show you how to score your answers and determine the best way to personalize your program. If you don't want to write in the book, go to my website, www. DrAliciaStanton.com, and download a copy of the quiz you can write on.

Part A

	Always	*Sometimes*	*Never*
I am often anxious and irritable.		X	
I am often depressed.		X	
I have a hard time falling asleep.		X	
I have breast pain and/or fibrocystic breast disease.		X	
I have heavy menses.			X
My menses are irregular.			X
I have a history of low thyroid.	X		
I have a lot of stress in my life.		X	
I have cervical dysplasia/abnormal Pap smears.			X
I am depressed or anxious.		X	
I have gained weight in my abdomen, hips, and thighs.	X		
I often retain water.		X	
I have uterine fibroids.			X
I am often fatigued.		X	
My diet is low in fiber.		X	
I have heart palpitations.		X	

Part B

	Always	*Sometimes*	*Never*
My skin is thinner and has more wrinkles.		✓	
My breasts have gotten smaller.			✓
I have urinary incontinence.			✓
My sex drive is decreased.			✓
My skin is oilier and/or I have acne.			✓
I am gaining belly fat.		✓	
I have vaginal dryness.		✓	
My memory is decreasing.		✓	
It is harder for me to stay asleep.		✓	
I am getting more urinary tract infections.			✓
My bone density is lower and/or I have osteoporosis.			✓
I am a smoker.			✓

Part C

	Always	*Sometimes*	*Never*
I am losing muscle mass even though I eat enough protein.		✓	✓
I am gaining weight.	✓		
I feel fatigue and low energy.	✓		
My self-confidence isn't what it used to be.	✓		
My sex drive is low.		✓	
I feel depressed.		✓	
I have muscle and joint pain.		✓	

	Always	Sometimes	Never
My skin is thin and dry.	___	_✗_	___
I feel anxious.	___	_✗_	___
My cholesterol is high.	___	___	_✗_
I have low bone mass and/or osteoporosis.	___	___	_✗_

Part D

	Always	Sometimes	Never
It is easy for me to catch colds.	___	___	_✗_
I am often irritable.	___	___	_✗_
I feel tired but wired.	___	___	_✗_
I crave sugar and sweets.	_✗_	___	___
It is hard for me to wind down and fall asleep at night.	___	_✗_	___
It is difficult for me to concentrate.	___	_✗_	___
It is easy for me to binge eat.	_✗_	___	___
I have night sweats.	___	___	_✗_
I am adding belly fat.	___	_✗_	___
I often feel stressed.	___	_✗_	___
My blood pressure is high.	___	_✗_	___
I have high cholesterol.	___	___	_✗_
My blood sugar is high.	___	_✗_	___
I am gaining weight.	___	_✗_	___
My skin bruises more easily.	___	___	_✗_

Part E

	Always	Sometimes	Never
I am exhausted no matter how much I sleep.		✕	
It is very difficult for me to wake up in the morning.		✕	
I am a disaster without caffeine in the morning.			✕
I get very sleepy at 3 or 4 o'clock in the afternoon.	✕		
I have digestive problems like diarrhea or constipation.			✕
I have low sexual interest.			✕
I get panic attacks or startle easily.			✕
I have sweaty hands and feet when I am nervous.			✕
I have mood swings.			✕
I am easily overwhelmed.			✕
I often feel weak or shaky.			✕
Bright light seems to bother me.			✕
I often wake up in the middle of the night.			✕
I get very cranky and shaky in between meals.			✕
It is very difficult to focus or concentrate.			✕
I do not have any motivation.			✕

Part F

	Always	*Sometimes*	*Never*
I am depressed.		X	
I have gained weight, and it is difficult to lose it.	X	X	
I am often constipated.			X
My skin is rough and dry.		X	
My menses are irregular.		X	
I am losing my hair.		X	
The outer third of my eyebrow has thinned out.		X	
I have muscle and joint pain/morning stiffness.		X	
My memory is poor.		X	
It is difficult to concentrate.		X	
My face is puffy, and my eyelids are often swollen.		X	
My hands and feet are often swollen.			X
My hands and feet are cold.			X
I am very tired.			X
I have a family history of thyroid problems.			X
My voice is hoarse.			X
I have carpal tunnel syndrome.			X
I have an autoimmune disease.			X
My body temperature is low.			X

Part G

	Always	*Sometimes*	*Never*
I crave sugar and carbohydrates.	✗		
I skip breakfast.			✗
I eat within two hours of going to bed.			✗
I eat fewer than three times a day.			✗
I eat high fructose corn syrup/ processed foods.			✗
I get less than eight hours of sleep at night.			✗
I eat fewer than five servings of fruits and vegetables a day.		✗	
I eat less than 30 grams of fiber a day.		✗	
I eat very little fat.		✗	

Part H

	Always	*Sometimes*	*Never*
I have gained weight.	✗		
I have increased belly fat.	✗		
I crave sweets and then "crash" about an hour after I eat them.	✗		
I get irritable and jittery between meals.	✗		
I eat very little fat.			✗
Once I start eating sweets, bread, or pasta, I cannot stop.	✗		
I cannot resist the bread basket.		✗	
It is difficult to concentrate.		✗	
I am calmer after eating.		✗	

	Always	Sometimes	Never
I get tired after eating.		X	
I am often very tired.		X	
I have a history of polycystic ovarian syndrome.			X
I have high blood pressure.		X	
I have chronic yeast infections/ jock itch.			X
I am often thirsty.			X
I have high cholesterol.			X
I have high blood sugar.			X

Part I

	Always	Sometimes	Never
I have a history of chronic infections (canker sores, cold sores).			X
I am exposed to pesticides and/or toxic chemicals.			X
I am exposed to heavy metals (machinist, dental office).			X
I get frequent colds and infections.			X
I have asthma or sinus problems.		X	
I have environmental or seasonal allergies.		X	
I have skin irritations like eczema or rashes.			X
I have arthritis.			X
I have an autoimmune disease.			X
I have irritable bowel syndrome.			X

	Always	*Sometimes*	*Never*
I exercise less than 30 minutes three times a week.		X	
I have food allergies.			X
I have a great deal of stress in my life.			X
I am overweight.	X		
I am sensitive to perfumes and smoke.	X		
I use tobacco products.			X
Someone in my home uses tobacco products.			X
I take prescription medications.	X	X	
I eat less than five servings of fruits and vegetables a day.		X	

Part J

	Always	*Sometimes*	*Never*
I am constipated.			X
I have mercury amalgams in my mouth.	X		
I eat swordfish, tuna, or shark more than once a week.	X		
I urinate small amounts of urine only a few times a day.			X
I have fibromyalgia.			X
I drink tap/well water.	X		
My clothes are dry cleaned.			X
I live in an urban or industrial area.			X

	Always	Sometimes	Never
I have had elevated liver enzymes.		X	
I have had jaundice (turned yellow).			X
I have a history of hepatitis.			X
I am bothered by perfumes, strong odors, smoke, etc.	X		
I regularly take Tylenol.			X
I regularly take acid-blocking drugs (Zantac, Pepcid, etc.).		X	
I regularly take birth control pills or hormones.			X
I regularly take ibuprofen or naproxen.		X	
I regularly take medications for chronic headaches.			X
I regularly take medications for allergy symptoms.		X	X
I regularly take medications for diarrhea.			X
I have food sensitivities.			X
I am often tired.		X	
I have chronic headaches.			X
I have muscle aches.			X

Scoring Your Quiz

For each question, score yourself 0 points for each "Never," 2 points for each "Sometimes," and 4 points for each "Always." Add the total number of points for each part so you can determine the areas where you need the most work. I give you suggestions and what your next steps should be based on the number of points you score in each part.

Part A—Low Progesterone/Estrogen Excess   Score: _28_

0–20: You're doing well! Follow the seven principles of the diet to maintain your balance.

22–42: There are definitely some concerns. Consider hormone testing to determine which of your hormones are out of balance. Focus on Principle #3 in Chapter 6.

44+: A hormone imbalance exists between estrogen and progesterone, which is creating a number of symptoms and will make it difficult for you to lose weight. You would definitely benefit from working with a physician who specializes in hormone imbalance. You should also consider hormone testing. Closely adhere to the seven principles and consider supplementation or hormone therapy, if indicated.

Part B—Low Estrogen   Score: _10_

0–14: You're doing well! Follow the seven principles of the diet to maintain your balance.

16–30: There are definitely some concerns. Consider hormone testing to determine which of your hormones are out of balance. Focus on Principle #3 in Chapter 6.

32+: A hormone imbalance exists due to low estrogen. One of estrogen's functions is to help your metabolism, so low estrogen might make it difficult for you to lose weight. You would definitely benefit from working with a physician who specializes in hormone imbalance. You should also consider hormone testing. Closely adhere to the seven principles and consider supplementation or hormone therapy, if indicated.

Part C—Low Testosterone   Score: _24_

0–12: You're doing well! Follow the seven principles of the diet to maintain your balance.

14–26: There are definitely some concerns. Consider hormone testing to determine which of your hormones are out of balance. Focus on Principle #3 in Chapter 6. Exercise and stress reduction are also known to increase testosterone naturally.

28+: You're definitely showing signs of low testosterone, which is creating a number of symptoms that will make it difficult for you to lose weight. I recommend that you find a physician who will work with you to evaluate your testosterone. You would benefit from hormone testing and closely adhering to the seven principles. Consider supplementation or hormone therapy, if indicated.

Part D—Elevated Cortisol   Score: _____22_____

0–18: You don't show a lot of signs of high cortisol. This is either because your corti-sol is balanced, or it might be too low. We can interpret this based on your symptoms and the results of Part E.

20–36: You're showing some signs of elevated cortisol, which will make it much more difficult for you to lose weight. Focus on Principle #4 in Chapter 7.

38+: You're very stressed! If you don't feel that you're emotionally stressed, there might be a hidden cortisol demand such as a food allergy or chronic infection. It will be extremely difficult, if not impossible, for you to lose weight with an elevated cortisol level. I recommend that you work with a physician who specializes in hor-mone imbalances. Consider a four-point salivary cortisol test with DHEA level (see Appendix B for the test) to see exactly what your adrenal function is. Focus on the stress reduction plans in Chapter 16, make sure you get enough sleep, and consider supplementation.

Part E—Low Cortisol   Score: _____8_____

0–20: You're not currently showing signs of low cortisol. This is either because your cortisol is balanced, or it might be too high. We can interpret this based in your symptoms and the results of Part D.

22–42: You're showing some signs and symptoms of low cortisol or adrenal fatigue. It will be more difficult to lose weight because your body has been stressed for such a long time that the metabolism is slower. Focus on the adrenal fatigue section in Chapter 16.

44+: You're showing signs of low cortisol or adrenal fatigue. I'll bet that you're really exhausted and having difficulty losing weight. I recommend that you do a four-point cortisol test and DHEA level to see how your adrenal function is (see Appendix B for testing recommendations). If you also show signs of low thyroid, make sure your adrenal glands are stable before you start any thyroid replacement. When you have low cortisol, you may not tolerate thyroid replacement well until your adrenal function has improved. Focus on the adrenal fatigue section in Chapter 16 and find a physician who can help you with supplementation of possible hormone therapy.

Part F—Low Thyroid   Score: _____22_____

0–22: You currently don't have signs of low thyroid function. Follow the seven prin-ciples to help you maintain optimal thyroid function.

24–48: You're showing some signs of low thyroid function. Because your thyroid is closely tied to your metabolism, it might be more difficult to lose weight. Thyroid is also closely tied to your cortisol levels. Be sure to focus on stress reduction and information in Chapters 7 and 16. You might want to consider asking your physician to order thyroid function testing and thyroid antibody testing (see the information at the end of the chapter).

50+: You may have a significant thyroid issue, which will lower your metabolism and make it very difficult to lose weight. I recommend consulting a physician to have your thyroid function and thyroid antibody tests done. You may also need to consider supplementation and thyroid therapy, if indicated. It's very important to remember that if you also have signs of low cortisol, you need to make sure that your cortisol levels and adrenal glands are stable prior to initiating any thyroid hormone therapy. If your cortisol levels are too low, you may not be able to tolerate thyroid therapy very well.

Part G—Appetite Regulation   Score: _____10_____

0–10: You're doing well! Continue to follow the seven principles to keep your appetite balanced.

12–22: If it's difficult to control your appetite, weight loss is more difficult. Focus on the information for Principle #6 in Chapter 9 and the action plans in Chapter 18.

24+: Appetite control may seriously hinder your ability to lose weight. Focus on Chapters 9 and 18. Also, I recommend you consult a physician and do some testing to determine whether a hormone imbalance is causing your increased appetite. Consider a two-hour blood sugar and insulin test to see whether you have metabolic syndrome.

Part H—High Insulin   Score: _____32_____

0–20: Your insulin level appears to be stable. Continue to follow the seven principles to maintain a healthy insulin level and metabolism.

22–42: You're showing signs of high insulin and may already be insulin resistant. Pay close attention to the information on insulin resistance in Chapter 1 and follow Principle #2 in Chapter 5 and the action plan in Chapter 13. Because it's easier to take care of this if it's caught early, I recommend consulting a physician and a lipid profile, fasting blood sugar, and fasting insulin test to check for insulin resistance.

44+: You're at high risk of being insulin resistant and may be prediabetic or diabetic at this point. In addition to following Chapters 5 and 13 closely, remember that stress and cortisol levels are also closely tied to insulin resistance. Also, inadequate sleep can contribute to insulin resistance. Focus on the information in Chapter 16 to help with sleep and stress reduction. Consult with your physician and consider a lipid profile, fasting blood sugar, fasting insulin, and two-hour blood sugar and insulin test. You may also want to consider supplementation to enhance your insulin sensitivity as well.

Part I—Inflammation   Score: _____ 20 _____

0–22: You're currently not showing significant signs of inflammation. Congratulations! Continue following the seven principles to keep your body in balance and reduce the risk of inflammation.

24–48: You're showing signs of general inflammation and may be at risk for chronic diseases if the inflammation continues. This also makes it more difficult to lose weight. Insulin resistance, adrenal fatigue, food intolerances, and chronic infections can all contribute to inflammation. You may want to consult a physician to help you address some of these potential causes of inflammation. You may also want to consider testing for the highly sensitive C-reactive protein homocysteine, have a complete blood count taken, and have your vitamin D level checked to see what your level of inflammation is.

50+: You have signs of significant inflammation and, in addition to having difficulty losing weight, are at risk for a number of chronic diseases. Consult a physician to help you test for and address potential insulin resistance, adrenal fatigue, gluten and food intolerances, infection, and toxin exposure. I recommend tests for the C-reactive protein homocysteine, a complete blood count, and a vitamin D level in addition to testing for insulin resistance. You should also consider supplementation with antioxidants and fish oils.

Part J—Detoxification   Score: _____ 24 _____

0–28: Your detoxification pathways appear to be functioning well, and you're limiting your exposure to toxins. Keep up the good work!

30–58: You may have some symptoms of poor detoxification and a possible increase in exposure to toxins. Remember, toxins are stored in your fat, so if you are not detoxifying well, it will be more difficult for you to lose fat. Focus on Principle #1 in Chapter 4 and the action plan in Chapter 12.

60+: You definitely have an increased exposure to toxins and a poor detoxification system. This will make it very difficult to lose weight. Also, since toxins are stored in fat, if you do lose fat, you will release the toxins and may not feel well. It's important to not only optimize your liver's ability to remove toxins but to reduce your exposure to toxins as well. Focus on the elimination of toxins and supplementation to enhance the function of your liver. Also, closely monitor your medications with your physician to make sure you're not adding undue stress to your liver.

Other Tests

A number of other tests can help you determine whether your health and metabolism are optimal. As you focus on the principles in this diet, you'll be able to watch the levels of your abnormal tests improve. These tests will help you know the function of your thyroid, liver, and detoxification system; insulin and blood sugar control system; energy production and metabolism; as well as the level of inflammation. You can download a copy of the list in the following table from my website, www. DrAliciaStanton.com, to take to your physician so the test can be ordered at your next physical exam.

Dr. Stanton's Recommended Optimal Laboratory Values

Laboratory Test	Recommended Level
Thyroid stimulating hormone (TSH)	Between 1.0 and 2.0
Free T3 and free T4	Mid-range for the lab
Thyroid antibodies	Negative
Fasting blood sugar	Less than 90 mg/dl
Fasting insulin	Less than 8 mIU/ml
Two-hour blood sugar test	Less than 120 mg/dl
Two-hour insulin test	Less than 30 mIU/ml
Highly sensitive C-reactive protein	Less than 1.0
Homocysteine	Less than 7.0
Vitamin D (25-hydroxy vitamin D)	50–80 ng/ml

Complete Blood Count

A complete blood count is one indicator of your general health. Your hemoglobin and hematocrit are measures related to your red blood cells and can tell your physician whether you're anemic or not. The red blood cells carry oxygen and, if they're low, you might be fatigued. This test also looks at your white blood cell count. Your white blood cells are important to help you fight infection and can be elevated (or very low) during an infection. Your platelet level, another part of this test, is one way to measure how well your blood will clot. Elevated platelets can also be a sign of inflammation.

Lipid Profile

Your lipid profile is another name for a cholesterol panel. Americans have become incredibly concerned about their levels of cholesterol. Everyone wants to know what their cholesterol "number" is. Television commercials and the majority of the medical community teach that the higher your cholesterol, the more likely you are to have a heart attack or stroke. However, the reality is that 50 percent of heart attacks occur in people with cholesterol levels less than 200, which is considered normal.

Many cholesterol abnormalities are caused by improper diet (refined carbohydrates, high fructose corn syrup, and trans fats) and hormone imbalance (low thyroid, low testosterone, and high insulin). Different functions of cholesterol include:

- Formation of hormones such as estrogen, progesterone, testosterone, DHEA, and cortisol

- Production of bile salts to aid in food digestion

- Conversion to vitamin D

- Production of the membranes around all cells

Cholesterol must get transported throughout your body in the bloodstream by being bound to protein because it's not soluble in your blood. The danger to your arteries is not necessarily cholesterol, but oxidized cholesterol. Remember, *oxidation* is caused by free radicals, and it's the same process as rust on metal. The real goal is to reduce the chance that you oxidize the cholesterol by limiting your exposure to free radicals and inflammation.

DEFINITION

Oxidation is the interaction between oxygen molecules and other substances. This is often seen as rust and the browning of an apple that has been cut in half.

The protein that carries cholesterol to the cells and tissues is called *low-density lipoprotein* (*LDL*), also known as the "bad" cholesterol. The protein that carries the cholesterol back to the liver is called *high-density lipoprotein* (*HDL*), also known as the "good" cholesterol. The ratio of bad cholesterol to good cholesterol is a better indicator of your risk for heart disease than the level of total cholesterol. Many physicians focus on this ratio now more than the level of total cholesterol. You can improve your ratio by eliminating refined carbohydrates, high fructose corn syrup, and trans fats.

Another substance measured in the lipid panel is *triglycerides*. Triglycerides are composed of free fatty acids and a glycerol molecule, and they're an excellent indirect measurement of insulin resistance. They are the chemical form in which most fat exists in the body and are a major component of very low-density lipoprotein or VLDL. Triglycerides also play an important role in metabolism as energy sources and transporters of dietary fat.

Elevated triglycerides are associated with a high intake of refined carbohydrates and high fructose corn syrup. In Chapter 1, you learned that excess sugar is converted into fat. To lower your triglyceride levels, eliminate refined carbohydrates, limit alcohol, increase your exercise, and make sure you're getting enough omega-3 fatty acids from foods or supplementation.

DEFINITION

Low-density lipoprotein (LDL) is a lipoprotein that enables lipids (fats) like cholesterol and triglycerides to be transported within the water-based bloodstream. It is referred to as "bad" cholesterol because higher levels of LDL are associated with increased heart disease.

High-density lipoprotein (HDL) is a lipoprotein made in the liver that transports cholesterol mostly back to the liver or organs such as adrenals, ovary, and testes, where steroid hormones are made. It is known as "good" cholesterol because it can remove cholesterol from arterial plaques for use in hormone production.

Triglycerides are made from glycerol and three fatty acids. They are the chemical form in which most fat exists in food as well as in the body.

Thyroid Function Tests

Thyroid function tests enable you to see how well your thyroid is working and, subsequently, how good your metabolism is. Many physicians look at only one measure of thyroid function: thyroid stimulating hormone or TSH. TSH actually comes from the pituitary gland and your brain to stimulate your thyroid gland. I often tell my patients that it's a measure of how hard your brain is yelling at your thyroid to work. So it's an indirect measure of how much thyroid hormone you actually have in your body. The higher the number is, the louder your brain is yelling at your thyroid to make thyroid hormone.

> **DID YOU KNOW?**
>
> Over the years, the upper limit of "normal" TSH has come down. Doctors used to think that your thyroid was "borderline low" or hypoactive if the TSH was between 5.0 and 10.0. In 2001, the American College of Endocrinologists suggested that the upper level of normal TSH should be 3.0. However, most laboratories and many doctors still look at the upper level of normal as being 5.0. This means that many people probably don't have optimal levels of thyroid hormone; you might even have symptoms of low thyroid, but because doctors are looking at the wrong reference ranges, you were told that your testing is "normal" and the thyroid is "fine."

It's also important for your physician to look at your free triiodothyronine (T3) and free thyroxine (T4) rather than total T3 or total T4. The total hormone levels represent the amount of hormone that is in your blood whether it is bound to a protein (not active) or not bound to a protein (active). Free hormone levels are the best measure of active thyroid hormone in your blood. Your thyroid secretes mostly T4, which has some activity. However, your body converts much of the T4 to another hormone, T3, which has five times more activity. That means the more T3 your body is able to make, the higher your metabolism and the easier it is to lose weight. Remember that stress, which causes high cortisol levels, significantly reduces your body's ability to convert T4 to T3. This is one of the reasons that it's hard to lose weight when you're stressed.

Thyroid Antibody Tests

Thyroid antibody tests look for antibodies against the thyroid created by your body in an autoimmune reaction. The antibodies can damage your thyroid and make it harder for it to work appropriately. I check for thyroid antibodies in my patients at least once a year to make sure that they're not damaging their thyroid. If one of my patients has antibodies against their thyroid, I suggest a gluten-free diet, fish oils, and antioxidants to reduce inflammation in the body. Very often, these suggestions work—the thyroid antibodies are reduced, the thyroid works much better, and their metabolism is increased.

Fasting Blood Sugar

Your fasting blood sugar is the measurement of your blood sugar first thing in the morning before you have anything to eat or drink. This is a good measure for your risk of diabetes. Please note that if you're insulin resistant, your fasting blood sugar might not yet be abnormal, but you're on a path toward diabetes and blood sugar elevation. You want your fasting blood sugar levels to be less than 90 mg/dl.

Fasting Insulin

Fasting insulin is the measurement of your insulin first thing in the morning before you have anything to eat or drink. It's a wonderful indicator for your risk of insulin resistance because it's elevated long before your blood sugar rises as a result of diabetes. Elevated fasting insulin tells you that your body is not listening well enough to a normal level of insulin and is becoming insulin resistant. This means your body has to produce more insulin. You want your fasting insulin level to be less than 8 mIU/ml.

Two-Hour Blood Sugar and Insulin Test

A two-hour insulin and blood sugar test is an excellent way to measure for insulin resistance and metabolic syndrome. This test is done by measuring a response to a 75-gram load of sugar. Usually, in order to make the test consistent, you consume a drink containing 75 grams of sugar (which is actually about what you find in two cans of soda). If your insulin response is elevated after two hours, it means that your body is not listening as well to insulin, and you need to produce a lot more than usual to keep your blood sugar stable. If your blood sugar response is elevated after two hours, it means that even with a higher level of insulin, you still can't keep your blood sugar under control, and you're at very high risk for diabetes. Your two-hour insulin level should be less than 30 mIU/ml, and your two-hour blood sugar level should be less than 120 mg/dl.

Highly Sensitive C-Reactive Protein

Inflammation is felt to be a major contributor to many other diseases that you might face, such as heart disease, diabetes, Alzheimer's, and cancer. It's an important part of your body's response to injury or infection. However, if left unchecked, chronic inflammation can create major problems.

The highly sensitive C-reactive protein is one of the best markers you have to measure inflammation throughout your body. C-reactive protein is a protein produced by your liver in response to inflammation. The normal level for highly sensitive C-reactive protein is less than 3.0. The optimal level is less than 1.0. It's important to know how much inflammation you have in your body. As you follow the principles of this diet, you'll reduce your level of inflammation and should see this number come down. If your number is greater than 1.0, follow the principles of this diet and add 3,000 milligrams of fish oil (EPA/DHA).

Homocysteine

Homocysteine is an amino acid found in the body and is involved in the production of the amino acid cysteine. However, this reaction depends heavily on some of the B vitamins (folic acid or B_9, B_6, and B_{12}), and if there are deficiencies in these vitamins, homocysteine levels can be elevated. High homocysteine levels have been associated with an increased risk of cardiovascular disease and fractures in the elderly. Because B vitamins are also incredibly important for optimal metabolism, monitoring your homocysteine level is a good way to make sure your B vitamin levels are adequate, and your risk for heart disease and fractures is low. I like to see the homocysteine level less than 7.0.

Vitamin D

Vitamin D has been found to help many functions, including increasing absorption of calcium and phosphorus to help with bone mineralization. Vitamin D deficiency has also been implicated in 16 varieties of cancer and other diseases, such as heart disease, diabetes, depression, and osteoporosis. Because vitamin D also helps the pancreas release insulin, adequate vitamin D levels are helpful for weight loss. I measure patients' vitamin D levels at least once a year and supplement with 2,000 to 5,000 IU per day depending on their levels. My goal is to have my patients reach a level of 25-hydroxyvitamin D between 50 and 80 ng/ml.

The Least You Need to Know

- There are many tests available to help determine whether your metabolism is running well.
- Many symptoms of hormone imbalance overlap, so it is often important to look at all the hormones to determine which ones are actually not balanced.
- If you have high levels of inflammation, it is difficult to lose weight, and you are at risk for chronic disease.
- It is just as important to limit your exposure to toxins as it is to support your liver so it functions well.

Energize with Less Stress and More Sleep

In This Chapter

- Understanding adrenal fatigue
- How to overcome adrenal fatigue
- Understanding the connection of adrenal fatigue and sleep
- Exploring options for stress reduction

Adrenal fatigue occurs when the adrenal glands can no longer produce enough of the stress hormone cortisol to adequately support many activities. It's often associated with significant prolonged stress. However, it can also arise after a series of smaller stressors that have a cumulative effect or after an acute or chronic infection, especially respiratory infections. With adrenal fatigue, the adrenal glands don't function well enough to support an active lifestyle.

This produces symptoms of extreme fatigue unrelieved by sleep, difficulty losing weight, and a host of other symptoms. Many people suffering from adrenal fatigue treat themselves by drinking coffee, soda, and caffeinated energy drinks to get the energy to push themselves through their days. In this chapter, I give you the information you need to understand and prevent adrenal fatigue.

When Your Adrenal Glands Are Exhausted

Because cortisol has so many effects on your body, if you have adrenal fatigue, or reduced cortisol output, it can cause significant problems. The adrenal glands mobilize your body's responses to every kind of stress (whether it's physical, emotional, or psychological) through hormones that regulate energy production and storage, immune function, heart rate, muscle tone, and other processes that enable you to cope with the stress.

As the amount of cortisol your adrenals are able to produce continues to fall, more and more systems in your body have problems. Changes occur with variations in your fluid and electrolyte balance, heart, and cardiovascular system. On top of that, your protein fat and carbohydrate metabolism is reduced, so it's more difficult to lose weight, and your sex drive might be reduced as well. Many other changes take place in your body in response to and to compensate for the decrease in cortisol that occurs with adrenal fatigue. Some people are so fatigued by the condition that they can't get out of bed for more than a few hours at a time. Your body does its best to make up for under-functioning adrenal glands, but it does so at a price. Adrenal fatigue can create a wide variety of symptoms.

Symptoms of adrenal fatigue include the following:

- Allergies

- Dizziness when standing quickly and headaches

- Easily frustrated, irritability, difficulty concentrating, and depression

- Fatigue

- Hypoglycemia

- Palpitations and panic attacks

- Poor memory

- Sugar, sweet, and salt cravings

- Weight gain

Common Causes of Adrenal Fatigue

In addition to stress, some potentially serious medical problems can cause adrenal fatigue. If you have sudden or persistent fatigue, contact your physician to make sure that you don't have another underlying medical problem. Medical causes of adrenal fatigue can include the following:

- **Anemia:** This blood disorder results from a number of problems that can reduce the number of red blood cells you have. Because the hemoglobin and red blood cells carry your oxygen, your blood's ability to transport oxygen is reduced, which causes fatigue.

- **Cancer:** Fatigue can be a symptom of cancer. A thorough checkup, including routine cancer screenings, can help rule out malignancy as a cause of your fatigue.

- **Chronic fatigue syndrome (CFS):** This is a complicated disorder characterized by extreme fatigue that doesn't improve with bed rest and might worsen with physical or mental activity. Of all chronic illnesses, CFS is one of the most mysterious and is often a diagnosis of exclusion. Severe and debilitating fatigue, muscle aches, and difficulty concentrating are the most commonly reported symptoms of CFS.

- **Depression:** This causes several symptoms, including sadness, loss of appetite, difficulty sleeping, a lack of interest in pleasurable activities, and difficulty concentrating. Talk to your doctor if you suffer from this group of symptoms.

- **Diabetes:** Extreme fatigue can be a warning sign of diabetes. Other signs and symptoms of diabetes, in addition to fatigue, include excessive thirst, frequent urination, blurred vision, and recurring infections.

- **Hypothyroidism:** This is a condition in which your thyroid gland fails to make or release enough thyroid hormone. Signs and symptoms include sluggishness, chronically cold hands and feet, constipation, dry skin, and a hoarse voice.

- **Medications:** Prescription or over-the-counter medications might cause fatigue or make you too restless to sleep well. Antihistamines, cough and cold remedies, some antidepressants, and many other drugs might make you tired. Talk to your doctor if you suspect your medications are making you tired.

- **Restless legs syndrome (RLS):** This condition is characterized by an inability to keep your legs still and by tingling or aching sensations in your legs, feet, or arms. The symptoms generally occur at night, preventing sound sleep.

- **Sleep apnea:** Signs of this disorder include loud snoring, pauses between breaths, and awakening frequently while gasping for air. It's a common source of fatigue because it interferes with sound sleep. Losing weight and quitting smoking might help, as well as an adjustment in sleeping position. Lying on your side or facedown might reduce snoring.

In addition to the many sources of stress that we are all familiar with, adrenal fatigue can result from a number of other situations that can create stress on the body. Other causes of adrenal fatigue follow.

- Chemical or environmental toxins

- Depression

- Emotional trauma

- Excess exercise

- Infections

- Insomnia/lack of sleep

- Poor nutrition

- Toxic relationship/work environment/home environment

Diagnosing Adrenal Fatigue

If you have the symptoms of adrenal fatigue listed previously, you should have your adrenal glands tested to see what your cortisol levels are. One of the best measurement tools for cortisol is saliva testing. Your saliva is a good indicator of what hormones are contained in the fluid around most of the cells in your body. Therefore, by getting a saliva sample, you can determine what your level of cortisol is at various points during the day. In fact, saliva cortisol testing is covered by Medicare Plan B. The National Institutes of Health and the World Health Organization recognize saliva cortisol testing as accurate. Some insurance plans also cover saliva cortisol testing.

The saliva cortisol test involves simply spitting into a test tube. Cortisol is measured four times—in the morning (8 A.M.), at noon, in the evening (4 P.M.), and at night (between 11 P.M. and midnight). Other steroid hormones, such as estrogen, progesterone, DHEAS, and testosterone, can be measured along with cortisol in the 8 A.M. saliva sample, if desired. You carry the test tubes with you during the day (they easily fit into a pocket or purse) so they are handy when it's time to give a saliva sample.

Treating Adrenal Fatigue

The mainstay of treatment for adrenal fatigue focuses on changes in diet and life-style habits. Most people develop adrenal fatigue after and during long periods of significant stress or multiple small stressors in a row. Therefore, it makes sense to do everything possible to reduce the sources of stress and your response to them.

This means eating in such a way that you maintain a stable blood sugar and reduce your cortisol demand. Also, it's imperative that you get enough rest and sleep. Your body needs at least eight to nine hours of uninterrupted sleep per night. It's well established that inadequate sleep upsets your insulin balance, which disturbs cortisol. But inadequate sleep in and of itself increases your demand for cortisol. In addition to getting adequate sleep, I recommend that my patients rest in between working hours so they're more refreshed and able to get through their work. Also, I suggest taking regular breaks from work and taking vacations.

TRUSTY TIP

Even if a patient can't afford to go away for vacation, I recommend taking a "stay-cation" during which they remain at home, take time to do things for themselves that they have been neglecting, and relax.

Good nutrition and stable blood sugar can heal adrenal fatigue. The principles of this diet will do just that. A diet that treats adrenal fatigue includes healthy proteins like poultry, fish, beef and beans, vegetables, high-fiber fruits, and nuts. In order to truly rest the adrenals, you have to completely avoid the consumption of chocolates, caffeine, processed and junk foods, refined sugars, and soft drinks.

In addition, your blood sugar will not remain stable if you skip meals. Therefore, you should build up the habit of eating regular healthy meals at least four to five times a day. If you have to get up early, eat breakfast by 8 A.M. or within an hour of getting up to restore blood sugar levels after using glycogen stores at night. Have a small mid-morning snack to keep blood sugar stable. Try to eat lunch between 11 A.M. and 1 P.M. because your morning meal can be used up quickly. Eat a nutritious snack between 2 and 3 P.M. to get you through the natural dip in cortisol around 3 or 4 P.M. Make an effort to eat dinner around 5 or 6 P.M., and make this your lightest meal of the day. Also, if you're addicted to cigarettes, alcohol, or drugs, it's crucial for you to stop them to effectively recover from adrenal fatigue.

Wide varieties of relaxation techniques are listed at the end of this chapter. Even if you don't usually have the time to relax, in order to heal your adrenals, you need to change your habits and make the time. Everyone has time to do something simple like practicing gratitude or deep breathing. Also, it's important to get some form of mild exercise to help reduce tensions and anxiety. Keep in mind, when you're healing from adrenal fatigue is not a time to start training for a marathon or any activity that involves too much exercise, because these things will only increase your cortisol demand. It's best to start with walking, swimming, or gentle bike riding until you begin to heal. Increase your activity level as you improve.

Dr. James Wilson wrote an excellent book called *Adrenal Fatigue*. I highly recommend it for anyone who has the symptoms and feels that they might be suffering from this syndrome. Unfortunately, although millions of people suffer from adrenal fatigue in the United States and around the world, many physicians don't appreciate its validity. I have seen hundreds of patients with adrenal fatigue, and I know for a fact that it exists. Many of these patients are told, "Your labs are fine" or "You're just getting old, get used to it." As more physicians understand and appreciate this syndrome, patients will get the right information on how to stop damaging their adrenal glands and start healing them.

In addition to diet, lifestyle changes, and stress reduction, supplementation might be helpful as you recover from adrenal fatigue. The supplements in the following tables are specific to help your adrenal glands heal and improve your energy. Some of the herbs such as ashwaganda, rhodiola, and ginseng are known as *adaptogens*. Adaptogens are thought to have a normalizing effect on the body and to be capable of either toning down or strengthening the activity of the endocrine and the immune systems. If you're on other medications, discuss these supplements with your physician before taking them.

DEFINITION

An **adaptogen** is an herb product that is thought to increase resistance to stress, trauma, anxiety, and fatigue.

General Adrenal Support Supplements

Supplement	Dose
Ashwaganda	160 mg twice a day
Cordyceps	400 mg twice a day
Ginseng	200 mg twice a day
Rhodiola	50 mg twice a day
Vitamin B_6	100 mg twice a day
Vitamin C	1,000 mg twice a day

Supplementation to Support Adrenals During Anxiety and Stress

Supplement	Dose
Ashwaganda	1,000 mg a day
B vitamin complex	100 mg each
Chromium	300 mg a day
Magnesium glycinate	600 mg at night

Supplementation to Support Adrenals If You're Fatigued

Supplement	Dose
Ashwaganda	1,000 mg a day
B complex	100 mg each
Cordyceps	400 mg twice a day
Ginseng	200 mg twice a day
Rhodiola	50 mg twice a day

Steps to Improve Your Sleep

Make sure your sleeping conditions support a good night's sleep. First, make sure the room is quiet enough because if you're woken up by a sound, it might disturb your sleep cycle and make it more difficult for you to fall back asleep. If you live in the city or can't get away from external noise, consider earplugs or an ambient noise machine.

Second, make sure that your room is an appropriate temperature, not too hot or too cold. Usually, it's recommended that you sleep in a cooler room. However, the most important thing is that you're comfortable enough to sleep.

Third, make sure your room is absolutely dark. Lights in your room—whether they're from your television, clock, computer, hall light, or any other source—disturb the production of melatonin, your sleep hormone. Cover your clock and any other light sources in your room during the night. Last, make sure your room is comfortable and inviting for sleep.

One of the most important things about getting a good night's sleep is making sure your blood sugar level stays stable throughout the night. If your blood sugar level drops during the night, your body interprets that as stress and releases your stress hormone, cortisol. The cortisol release wakes you up and then you may have a hard time falling back to sleep. Make sure you're not eating refined sugars or drinking beverages with caffeine, especially close to bedtime. Also, although you might think alcohol relaxes you and helps you to fall asleep more easily, it actually creates a drop in blood sugar during the middle of the night, and the corresponding stress hormone release wakes you up.

Before you go to sleep, set yourself up to get a good night's rest. Try to do something relaxing like reading, meditating, or taking a warm bath before bed. If you're doing chores, sitting on the computer, or having an emotionally charged discussion, you'll raise your cortisol level and it'll be more difficult for you to fall asleep. If you find the need to get up during the night to urinate, take a close look at how much fluid you drink in the evening. If you don't drink a lot of fluid but still have to get up to urinate, speak to your physician to make sure you don't have a problem with your bladder or diabetes.

Melatonin is a hormone secreted naturally by the pineal gland. It is the sleep hormone and is said to induce sleep without any negative side effects. Melatonin is found naturally in plants and in algae. In several studies, supplementation with melatonin has been found to be helpful in inducing and maintaining sleep for both people with normal sleep patterns and those suffering from insomnia. It's also useful in banishing jet lag. However, it appears that the sleep-promoting effects of melatonin are most apparent only if a person's melatonin levels are low. In other words, taking melatonin is not like taking a sleeping pill or even 5-HTP. It will only produce a sedative effect when melatonin levels are low. Melatonin appears to be most effective in treating insomnia in the elderly, as low melatonin levels are common in this age group. I usually have my patients start at 1 milligram 30 to 45 minutes before bed.

Don't take a melatonin supplement if …

- You are pregnant or breast-feeding.
- You are suffering from cancer of the blood or immune system.
- You have kidney disease.

5-HTP provides an effective, consistent result in treating insomnia. It's an effective alternative for dealing with sleep problems in a safe and natural way compared to sleep medicines. 5-HTP improves the quality of sleep and increases REM sleep significantly (typically by about 25 percent) while simultaneously increasing deep-sleep stages III and IV without increasing total sleep time. 5-HTP accomplishes this by shortening the amount of time you spend in sleep stages I and II, which in certain ways are the least important stages of the cycle. The higher the dose, the more time spent in REM. By shifting the balance of the sleep cycle, 5-HTP can make sleep more restful and rejuvenating.

The impact of 5-HTP on sleep stages is dose-related; taking higher doses produces a somewhat greater impact. In most cases, the lower dosage is adequate. Higher doses may lead to a greater number of disturbing dreams and nightmares due to abnormally prolonged REM sleep. It can also lead to mild nausea. I recommend starting with the lowest dose, 50 milligrams, about 30 to 45 minutes prior to going to bed.

The following table lists supplements for sleep.

Supplements for Sleep (Buy Pharmaceutical Grade)

Supplement	Dose
5-HTP	50–200 mg at night
GABA	300–500 mg at night
Inositol	1,000–2,000 mg at night
Magnesium glycinate	600 mg at night
Melatonin	1–3 mg at night (best for jet lag)

Know Your Sources of Stress

One of the first things you need to do when you begin thinking about stress management or stress reduction is to appreciate what creates stress in your life. One way to do this is to get out a piece of paper and write headings that correlate with various aspects of your life: your home life, your job, your family, your relationships, your hobbies, and so on. Under each heading, write down the things that create stress for you—whether it's your boss, your commute, not feeling satisfied at work, a family issue, or any number of other things.

Stress Reduction Techniques

You can't avoid all stress, but you can counteract its negative effects by learning how to relax—a state of deep rest is the opposite of the stress response. The stress response floods your body with chemicals that prepare you for fight or flight. But although the stress response is helpful in true emergency situations in which you must be alert, it wears down your body when constantly activated. Relaxation brings your system back into balance: deepening your breathing, reducing stress hormones, slowing down your heart rate and blood pressure, and relaxing your muscles.

In addition to its calming physical effects, research shows that relaxing also increases energy and focus, combats illness, relieves aches and pains, heightens problem-solving abilities, and boosts motivation and productivity. Best of all, a variety of relaxation techniques exist; there's something for everyone.

Those whose stress-busting benefits have been widely studied include deep breathing, progressive muscle relaxation, meditation, visualization, yoga, and tai chi. Learning the basics of these relaxation techniques isn't difficult. However, it takes time and daily practice to truly harness their stress-relieving power. Most experts recommend at least 10 to 20 minutes a day for your relaxation practice. If you'd like to get even more stress relief, aim for 30 minutes to an hour.

The best way to start and maintain a relaxation practice is by incorporating it into your daily routine. Schedule a set time either once or twice a day for your practice. You might find that it's easier to stick with your practice if you do it first thing in the morning, before other tasks and responsibilities get in the way. Don't practice when you're sleepy. These techniques can relax you so much that they can make you very sleepy, especially if it's close to bedtime. You'll get the most out of these techniques if you practice when you're fully awake and alert.

Choose a technique that appeals to you. No single relaxation technique is best for everyone. When choosing a relaxation technique, consider your specific needs, preferences, and fitness level. The right relaxation technique is the one that resonates with you and fits your lifestyle. If you crave solitude, solo relaxation techniques such as meditation or progressive muscle relaxation will give you the capability to quiet your mind and recharge your batteries. If you crave social interaction, a class setting will give you the stimulation and support you're looking for. Practicing with others might also help you stay motivated.

Deep Breathing

Stress causes rapid, shallow breathing. If you slow down and deepen your breathing, you can reduce the effects of stress. With its focus on full, cleansing breaths, deep breathing is a simple yet powerful relaxation technique. It's easy to learn, can be practiced almost anywhere, and provides a quick way to get your stress levels in check. Deep breathing is the cornerstone of many other relaxation practices, too, and can be combined with other relaxing elements such as aromatherapy and music. All you really need is a few minutes and a place to stretch out.

The key to deep breathing is to breathe deeply from the abdomen, getting as much fresh air as possible in your lungs. When you take deep breaths from the abdomen, rather than shallow breaths from your upper chest, you inhale more oxygen. The more oxygen you get, the less tense, short of breath, and anxious you feel. So the next time you feel stressed, take a minute to slow down and breathe deeply by following these steps:

1. Sit comfortably with your back straight. Put one hand on your chest and the other on your stomach.

2. Breathe in through your nose. Inhale. With your mouth closed and your shoulders relaxed, inhale as slowly and deeply as you can, to the count of six. At the same time, push your stomach out. Allow the air to fill your diaphragm. The hand on your stomach should rise. The hand on your chest should move very little. Inhale.

3. Hold. Keep the air in your lungs as you slowly count to four.

4. Exhale. Release the air through your mouth as you slowly count to six, pushing out as much air as you can while contracting your abdominal muscles. The hand on your stomach should move in as you exhale, but your other hand should move very little.

5. Repeat. Complete the inhale-hold-exhale cycle three to five times. Continue to breathe in through your nose and out through your mouth. Try to inhale enough so that your lower abdomen rises and falls. Count slowly as you exhale.

If you have a hard time breathing from your abdomen while sitting up, try lying on the floor. Put a small book on your stomach and try to breathe so that the book rises as you inhale and falls as you exhale.

Meditation

Meditation is a group of techniques rooted in spiritual traditions. Many people use meditation for stress and pain reduction and to promote wellness. When meditating, you use one of a range of techniques, such as repeating a word over and over again (a mantra) or paying attention to your breathing. These approaches help focus your attention and quiet down your stress-related thoughts. No one really knows how it works, but for many people, meditation leads to physical relaxation, pain reduction, and psychological balance. A number of guided meditation CDs are available on the market. However, you can meditate on your own at home very easily as well.

A few simple steps will make meditation easy enough for anyone to try. Make sure you use a quiet location with few distractions, and keep your posture comfortable. Focus your attention on only one thing. Many people use a simple mantra or a picture that is special to them. Don't get too frustrated if you find that your mind wanders; it happens to everyone early on. Simply acknowledge that your mind has wandered (without beating yourself up) and focus your attention back on your focal point (mantra or picture).

Here's a sample meditation exercise to try at home. Find a peaceful place where you'll be free of interruptions. Choose a focus word, a phrase, or an image you find relaxing. Examples of words are "grace" and "ooohmmm." (Some practitioners believe that the mantra should be syllables or words that have no meaning to you. That is why many people use "ooohmmm" or "aaaaummm.") Examples of phrases you can use are "May I be well," or "May I have patience and gratitude." Examples of images to concentrate on include a statue of a spiritual figure or a photograph of the sun.

1. Sit quietly in a comfortable position. The easiest posture is a comfortable sitting position, with your spine straight and erect. If you lie down, you'll probably fall asleep, and you can't meditate when you're unconscious!

2. Close your eyes and relax your muscles, starting at your head and working down your body to your feet.

3. Breathe slowly and naturally, focusing on your word, phrase, or image. Continue for 10 to 20 minutes. If your mind wanders, that's okay. Gently return your focus to your breathing and to the word, phrase, or image you've previously selected.

4. After the time is up, sit quietly for a few minutes with your eyes closed. Open your eyes and sit in silence for a few more minutes.

Guided Imagery

Guided imagery can help you use your imagination to calm the stress that reality brings to your life every day. This technique involves creating positive images, sounds, smells, tastes, and feelings with your mind. An instructor—in person or on audiotape—guides you through the process of forming your own imagery. One commonly used technique is to imagine a safe, comfortable place such as a beach on a pleasant, clear day or a peaceful chapel in the autumn woods.

Guided imagery is frequently used in hospital settings due to the success of a study conducted at the Cleveland Clinic in the mid-1990s. Clinic researchers found that employing guided imagery reduced their patients' anxiety and pain, as well as their use of narcotic medication both before and after surgery.

> **DID YOU KNOW?**
>
> The technique of guided imagery has become so popular that Kaiser Permanente, a major health maintenance organization, provides patients and the public with free downloads of guided imagery to use during medical procedures and for overall wellness at http://members.kaiserpermanente. org/redirects/listen. Guided imagery tapes are also widely available through bookstores and the web.

Gratitude Journal

It's impossible to feel stress and gratitude at the same time. A gratitude journal is an excellent way for you to clearly see the many things you have to be grateful for. Any kind of notebook or journal works. However, it's important that you write in it only what you're grateful for and do so every day. Many people choose the morning to write in their journals because they feel it gets their day off to a good start. No matter what your situation is, you can always find something to be grateful for, such as:

- The fact that you are alive
- Beautiful sunsets
- A baby's laugh
- A stranger's smile
- Shoes on your feet

When you stop focusing on what you don't have and start focusing on what you have, you'll immediately feel more peaceful. That's the beginning of your attitude of gratitude. As you continue to write in your gratitude journal, the attitude of gratitude becomes natural to you, and you'll experience less stress in your life and more freedom.

You don't have to write in your journal in any specific way. You can write long, descriptive paragraphs about your activities of the day and what you appreciated about them. You can make a journal that just lists the things you're grateful for. Or you can choose a preset number or leave it open to write as much or as little as you want that day. Your main goal is to be in a state of mind that reflects gratitude.

The best way to be successful in keeping a journal is to create a schedule and stick to it. The more often you write in your journal, the more likely you are to continue doing so. Try to find a consistent time each day that works best for your schedule. You can begin each day writing in it or make it the last thing you do at night. At first, it might be hard to keep this commitment because everyone has a million other things they could be doing. However, it's important to keep your commitment to yourself because, in the long run, it will make you better able to keep commitments to others.

In addition to keeping the journal, frequently remind yourself to be grateful through-out your day. Find yourself a small gratitude object that you can carry in your pocket or in your purse. It can be a small rock, a talisman, or anything that you associate with gratitude. Every time you hold or look at your gratitude object, it will remind you to be grateful for what you have and to think about things you write in your journal every day. You'll naturally begin to look for something to be thankful for. When you develop an attitude of gratitude, your whole being will radiate. And you'll experience more peace, joy, and happiness in life.

Having a reminder to be grateful will make it easier to catch yourself when you aren't in a positive state. Quite often, people go about their days and don't realize that they're feeling stressed out, depressed, or annoyed. Being aware of your feelings is an important step toward your well-being. Stop frequently throughout the day and ask yourself how you're feeling. If you aren't feeling good, then change it. How? Begin to count your blessings.

Most importantly, remember that all your gratitude doesn't need to be saved for just you. You can try to be vocal about your appreciation. If you tell people in your family how much you appreciate them or tell that sales clerk that you like the job he's doing, you might make all the difference in the world to them. If they can see their good-ness through your eyes, they will really appreciate you, and their reactions will leave you feeling positive, too.

Yoga

Dating back more than 5,000 years, yoga is the oldest defined practice of self-development. The methods of classical yoga include ethical disciplines, physical postures, breathing control, and meditation. Traditionally an Eastern practice, it's now becoming popular in the West. In fact, many companies, especially in Britain, see the benefit of yoga and are sponsoring yoga fitness programs.

Many of the popular techniques found to reduce stress are derived from yoga: controlled breathing, meditation, physical movement, mental imagery, and stretching.

Yoga—which derives its name from the word *yoke*, "to bring together"—does just that, bringing together the mind, body, and spirit. But whether you use yoga for spiritual transformation or for stress management and physical well-being, the benefits are numerous and include the following:

- Reduced stress and reduced cortisol levels
- Sound sleep
- Improvement of many medical conditions
- Allergy and asthma symptom relief
- Lower blood pressure and lower heart rate
- Smoking cessation help
- Spiritual growth
- Sense of well-being
- Reduced anxiety and muscle tension
- Increased strength and flexibility
- Slowed aging process

The practice of yoga involves stretching the body and forming different poses while keeping breathing slow and controlled. The body becomes relaxed and energized at the same time. Various styles of yoga exist, some moving through the poses more quickly, almost like an aerobic workout, and other styles relaxing deeply into each pose. Some have a more spiritual angle, and others are used purely as a form of exercise.

Tai Chi

Tai chi is translated as "the ultimate" and its theory and practice evolved in agreement with many Chinese philosophical principles, including those of Taoism and Confucianism. Although the image of tai chi chuan in popular culture is typified by exceedingly slow movement, many tai chi styles have secondary forms at a faster pace. Some traditional schools of tai chi teach partner exercises known as "pushing hands" and martial applications of the forms' postures.

Since the first widespread promotion of tai chi's health benefits, it has developed a worldwide following among people with little or no interest in martial training, for its benefit to health and health maintenance. Medical studies of tai chi support its effectiveness as an alternative exercise and a form of martial arts therapy. It's purported that focusing the mind solely on the movements of the form helps to bring about a state of mental calm and clarity. Many general health and stress management benefits are attributed to tai chi training.

The physical techniques of tai chi chuan are described in the tai chi classics (classical texts used as guides for the practice of the Chinese martial art of tai chi) as being characterized by the use of leverage through the joints based on coordination and relaxation, rather than muscular tension, in order to neutralize or initiate attacks. The slow, repetitive work involved in the process of learning how that leverage is generated gently and measurably increases the internal circulation (breath, body heat, blood, lymph, peristalsis, and so on).

The study of tai chi chuan primarily involves three aspects:

- **Health:** Tai chi's health training concentrates on relieving the physical effects of stress on the body and mind. For those focused on tai chi's martial application, good physical fitness is an important step toward effective self-defense.

- **Meditation:** The focus and calmness cultivated by the meditative aspect of tai chi is seen as necessary in maintaining optimum health (in the sense of relieving stress and maintaining homeostasis).

- **Martial art:** The ability to use tai chi as a form of self-defense in combat is the test of a student's understanding of the art. Tai chi chuan is the study of appropriate change in response to outside forces, the study of yielding and sticking to an incoming attack rather than attempting to meet it with opposing force.

Time for Yourself

When you get stressed, it's often important to find time for yourself. Solitude gives you a chance to reflect about your current situation and allow the options you have to become clearer. Consider that Buddha and Jesus both took the time for self-reflection before they felt capable of achieving their goals and guiding others. Your body and spirit both need nurturing, and time for yourself enables you to reduce the stress and nurture all aspects of yourself. In solitude, you can listen to the true "inner you" and discover that you're stronger than you think.

One of the best things about solitude and time for yourself is that you have the freedom to do what you desire—read for as long as you want, take a long bath, listen to your favorite music, go for a walk, take a nap, or just do nothing.

Humor

Laughter enhances the blood flow to the body's extremities and improves cardiovascular function. Laughter releases endorphins and other natural mood-elevating and pain-killing chemicals, and improves the transfer of oxygen and nutrients to internal organs. Laughter boosts the immune system and helps the body fight off disease; cancer cells; and viral, bacterial, and other infections.

In 1992, it was reported in *Health Progress* by Dr Brian Seaward in his article "Humor's Healing Potential" that the medical world has begun to take more serious the healing power of humor and the positive emotions associated with it. Humor and laughter are used by health-care professionals to promote and maintain health, as well as intervention for illnesses related to stress and lifestyle. Dr. Seaward states, "Laughter has many clinical benefits, promoting beneficial physiological changes and an overall sense of well-being. Humor even has long-term effects that strengthen the effectiveness of the immune system. In health care, humor therapy can help relieve stress associated with disease."

Progressive Muscle Relaxation

Progressive muscle relaxation (PMR) is a technique for reducing anxiety by alternately tensing and relaxing the muscles. It was developed by the American physician Edmund Jacobson in the early 1920s. He thought that since muscle tension accompanies anxiety, one can reduce anxiety by learning how to relax the muscles. PMR has both a physical and mental component.

The physical component involves the tensing and relaxing of muscle groups over the legs, abdomen, chest, arms, and face. With the eyes closed and in a sequential pattern, a given muscle group is purposefully tensed for about 10 seconds and then released for about 20 seconds before continuing to the next muscle group.

The mental component focuses on the difference between the feelings of tension and relaxation. Because the eyes are closed, you're forced to concentrate on the sensation of tension and relaxation. Simply focus on the feelings of the tensed muscle. Because the feelings of warmth and heaviness are felt in the relaxed muscle after it is tensed, a mental relaxation is felt as a result. With practice, you can learn how to effectively relax and reduce stress and anxiety when it reaches an unhealthy level.

Massage

Massage therapy with a professional massage therapist is a wonderful way to reduce stress. In addition, massage increases blood flow and the flow of lymphatic fluid through your body and is helpful for detoxification. But what if you don't have the time or money to see a massage therapist? Self-massage is a great option at these times. The idea behind self-massage is to rub and stroke the areas on your body that a massage therapist would stroke, and to concentrate on the areas that are showing the most signs of stress and pain. You probably do some of this without even thinking about it—rubbing your head when you have a headache, stroking your shoulders after hunching over a keyboard all day, or massaging your sore feet after a long hike.

The Least You Need to Know

- Adrenal fatigue can be caused by a long-term major stressor or a series of small stressors in a row.
- Diet and lifestyle changes are two important ways to help recover from adrenal fatigue.
- A wide variety of stress reduction techniques are available, which will suit any personality or any schedule.
- Laughter, deep breathing, and gratitude are examples of stress-reduction methods that can be practiced anywhere at any time.

Exercise and Interval Training

In This Chapter

- Aerobic versus anaerobic exercises
- Strength and interval training
- Step-by-step instructions for functional movement exercises

Like many people, you might equate exercise training with rows of treadmills, stationary bikes, and other equipment. And in most of the gyms and exercise clubs that are stocked with such equipment, you're usually encouraged to alternate 30 to 40 minutes of cardio with strength-training sessions utilizing isolated movements like lateral raises, leg extensions, and curls. However, studies show that interval training and strength training using complex, functional movements provide better fitness and result in better hormone profiles. This chapter gives you information on how to start an interval training program if you're a beginner and maintain a balanced program if you're more experienced.

Types of Interval Training

A *functional movement* mimics the nerve and muscle patterns that you use in everyday life. For example, the exercise called "squatting" is standing from a seated position; "dead lifting" is taking anything off the ground; and "the burpee" is lying all the way down on the ground and getting back up. Therefore, they are functional exercises. On the other hand, some of the isolation movements, such as leg extensions and leg curls, are nonfunctional exercises.

There are two important aspects of functional movements. First, they're mechanically sound, so they're safe. They're actions that you do every day, but you want to make sure that you do them in the safest and most effective way possible. Second, they create a high neuroendocrine response. This means that they help boost the hormones that you want boosted, such as testosterone and natural human growth hormone (HGH).

Aerobic training is an important part of any exercise regimen because it increases the oxygen supply to many of the tissues in your body, which then become more efficient at utilizing it. When oxygen consumption is increased, energy is made by burning calories. This is one of the ways you can lose weight.

There are many forms of aerobic exercise. Essentially, anything you do that increases your rate of breathing and your heart rate is aerobic because it increases oxygen demand. One way to ramp up your aerobic fitness is to utilize *interval training*.

You need to use both aerobic and *anaerobic* pathways to get your energy level where it needs to be when you do any kind of exercise. When you do exercises that are moderate to high power and that last less than several minutes, you use anaerobic (without oxygen) energy. When you do work at low power that lasts longer than several minutes, you use aerobic (with oxygen) energy.

DEFINITION

Functional movements are exercises that mimic the nerve and muscle patterns that you use in everyday life.

Aerobic actions increase your rate of breathing and demand for oxygen.

Interval training involves short periods of all-out effort followed by periods of lighter activity.

Anaerobic exercise is short-lasting, high-intensity activity, where your body's demand for oxygen exceeds the oxygen supply available. Anaerobic exercise relies on energy sources that are stored in the muscles and, unlike aerobic exercise, is not dependent on oxygen from (breathing) the air.

Aerobic training is beneficial for cardiovascular function and decreased body fat. It allows you to do low-power work over a longer period of time, more efficiently giving you endurance and stamina. This is important in many sports. However, if you were training only for increased aerobic capacity, you'd see a decrease in muscle mass, strength, speed, and power. Think of the body type of a marathoner: extremely lean with minimal muscle mass. Long-distance and ultra-endurance running, cross-country skiing, and 1500+-meter swimming are sports that require extensive aerobic training.

Anaerobic training also benefits cardiovascular function and decreases body fat. Even more interesting, anaerobic activity decreases body fat even better than aerobic activity! In addition, it can improve power, speed, strength, and muscle mass. This is true because anaerobic conditioning lets you exert much greater force over short time intervals. You're doing exercises at a level that you could not sustain longer than a few minutes. When done appropriately, anaerobic training can actually be used to develop a high level of aerobic fitness without the high volumes of aerobic exercise. This is the reason why anaerobic activity is so effective.

TRUSTY TIP

Be sure to keep a record of the exercises you do and how you score, so that you can keep track of your progress. You'll be able to see how you went from beginner to intermediate to advanced moves and how you were able to increase the number of exercises you do. Also, keep track of how you felt when you did the exercises and if you were sore a day or two after.

Make sure that you have "rest days" to give your body a chance to recover. Working out three days in a row followed by a "rest day" works best for me. However, you should figure out what works best for you.

Continuous Aerobic Exercise

If you're training in an endurance sport such as running, biking, rowing, or swimming, you will need to do some longer sessions of continuous aerobic activity. Keep in mind that your intensity will not be as high as what you could maintain over short intervals. Also, if walking is an easy thing for you to do, go right ahead. I don't want to discourage you from doing any continuous aerobic exercise if that is all you really have access to. However, I suggest that you try to incorporate the benefits of interval training as well.

Strength Training

Rather than focusing on isolation movements of specific muscles, researchers have shown that using groups of muscles in functional movements does a much better job. If you combine them with high-intensity aerobic and anaerobic cardiovascular workouts, the effect is even better.

In reality, everyone's physical fitness needs are all the same. Everyone needs strength, stamina, balance, coordination, and endurance, whether they're an elite athlete, a middle-aged mom, or a grandfather. Individuals need different degrees of each of them, including the elderly. You might not necessarily think of older people as needing strength training. But more and more research points to the fact that even a minimal training program can increase their strength and balance, leading to fewer falls and better general health overall.

Imagine if you entered your golden years with a fit, muscular body. Your risk of falls and fractures would be greatly decreased. Your bones and your heart would be strong. And the possibility that you would need assisted living would be much lower.

In general, athletes have better bone density, stronger immune systems, less coronary artery disease, less depression, reduced risk of cancer, and reduced risk of strokes than nonathletes. It doesn't matter if those athletes are 80 years old or 25 years old. I often say to my patients, "Remember, what you do today matters tomorrow." That is the truth about so many things, especially exercise.

This is the bottom line: you can begin strength training at any age and you'll get a benefit. However, the earlier you start, the longer you'll have the benefit.

Getting Smart with Dumbbells

It's easy to incorporate dumbbells into your workout. They're easy to use, effective at building your muscles, and can be used in a variety of ways. You'll be able to see in the upcoming workout section how the addition of dumbbells can increase the intensity of your workout. This reduces the risk of having your body plateau because it's no longer challenged by a given workout. For a minimal investment, you can purchase a small set of dumbbells and increase the variety of your exercises exponentially.

In addition, if you choose, you can get a few other basic pieces of exercise equipment to add more variety. Kettle bells come in a variety of weights, and you can use them in some of the exercises shown in this chapter. A jump rope also provides an excellent overall exercise and is portable, so you can travel with it.

Basic Movements

The following sections demonstrate the basic moves you should incorporate into your training.

The Squat

The squat is one of our most essential functional moves. As a matter of fact, the squat, in the bottom position, is the original way you were intended to sit (not in chairs), and the rise in the bottom of the squat to standing position is the way your body was intended to rise off the ground. Most of the world's populations don't sit in chairs. They sit in a squatting position for their meals, conversations, and ceremonies. In the industrialized world, Americans use chairs and couches, which has resulted in many of us losing functionality and increasing the weakness of major lower body and core muscle groups.

You may have been told by a doctor or chiropractor that the squat is dangerous. However, it's the basic movement necessary to get off the toilet or the floor. The squat is the most important hip extension exercise, and hip extension is a foundation for good movement. The squat also elicits a strong neuroendocrine response. After you master the air squat, you will add weights to increase the intensity.

1. Stand upright and start with feet about shoulder width apart and toes slightly turned out. Keep your head up. If this is new to you, start with a chair or box behind you. As you get better, make the level of the chair or box lower until you don't need it anymore. Basically, you want to just sit down, but you want to do so with excellent form.

2. Keep your midsection very tight. Set your butt back and down keeping your weight in your heels and making sure that your knees track over the line of your foot. Don't let your knees roll inside of your foot and stay off the balls of your feet. As you're descending, lift your arms out and up for counterbalance. Instead of just sinking, pull yourself down with your hip flexors. Stop when the fold of your hip is beneath your knee or you break the parallel with your thigh.

3. Squeeze your butt and the backs of your legs (glutes and hamstrings) and rise without leaning forward or shifting imbalance. Basically, you're reversing the process of going down, keeping your weight in your heels and your knees over your toes. Stand as tall as you possibly can with your hips back under your shoulders.

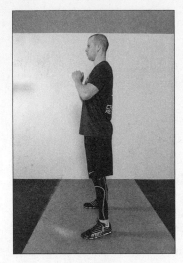
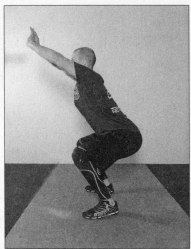
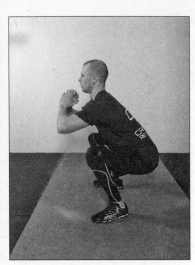

Squat.

This movement will increase the intensity of your squat: Lift a pair of dumbbells to your shoulders and perform your normal squat. Keep your core muscles tight, especially those of the stomach, back, and legs. Breathe at the top of each squat. Keep your elbows high; if your elbows drop, your back will round.

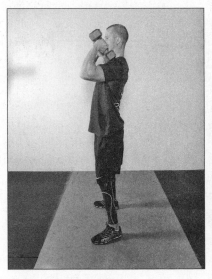
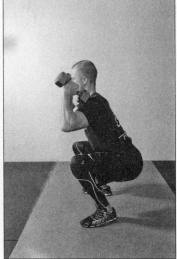

Front squat with dumbbells.

Pushups

Pushups are excellent for upper body strength. They can be modified to vary in intensity to allow for anyone, regardless of athletic ability, to start building their upper body strength. As you increase your strength, you can scale them up and progress to more difficult versions.

Wall Pushups

The wall pushup is the easy way to do a pushup:

1. Stand facing the wall a few inches away. Put your hands flat against the wall at a level just below your shoulders.

2. Step back a few inches and tighten your legs, stomach, and butt.

3. Push yourself away from the wall, extending your arms all the way.

4. Bend your arms and, in a slow and controlled fashion, lower yourself back down so that you're in starting position. Do not lock your elbows. Repeat this process. You can modify this pushup by moving your feet a little farther away from the wall to make it harder.

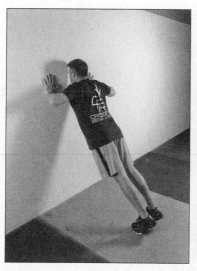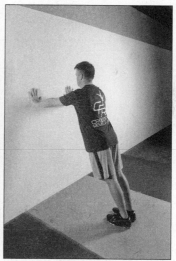

Wall pushup.

Knee Pushups

The knee pushup is another variation. You can choose to do this before or after the chair pushup.

1. Kneel on all fours with your arms straight and shoulder width apart in line with your shoulders and your fingers facing forward. Your knees should be under your hips.

2. Walk your hands out for about 6 inches and then press your hips forward until your body forms a straight line from your head to your hips. Tighten your abdominal muscles and squeeze your shoulder blades together. Keep your head neutral; you do not want to drop your chin and have your head tilt forward.

3. With your body tight, bend your elbows out to the side and lower your torso until your elbows are aligned with your shoulders.

4. Contracting your chest and your triceps, straighten your arms and return to the starting position. Do not lock your elbows.

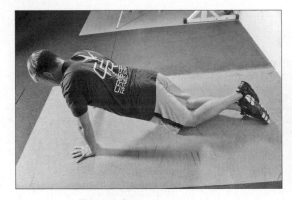 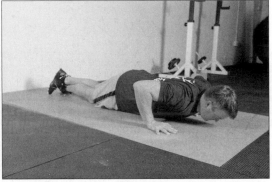

Knee pushup.

Chair Pushups

The chair pushup is a slightly harder variation you can try after you've mastered the wall pushup and the knee pushup. You're working against more of your bodyweight than you were with the wall.

1. Find a secure chair or box to start with. Stand next to the chair with your feet under your hips and place your hands securely on the seat of the chair or the box about shoulder width apart.

2. Walk your feet back until the lower portion of your ribs is touching the seat.

3. Tighten your legs, butt, and stomach and push yourself off the chair, fully extending your arms.

4. Keeping your body tight, slowly lower yourself back to your starting position. Do not lock your elbows.

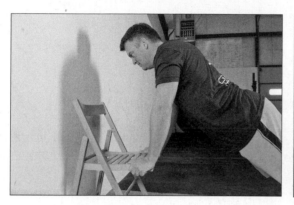 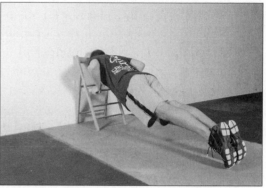

Chair pushup.

Full Pushups

Full pushups are a more difficult variation than the chair pushup. At this point, you're working against your entire bodyweight. Make sure you focus on your form!

1. Start by kneeling on all fours, your arms slightly more than shoulder width apart and your fingers facing forward.

2. Contract your abdominal muscles and extend one leg at a time behind you so that you're supported on the balls of your feet. Your body should form a straight line from your head to your heels. Look straight down, keeping your head in a neutral position.

3. Maintaining your starting position, bend your elbows out to the side. Lower your torso toward the floor with your elbows bent at 90-degree angles in line with your shoulders.

4. Contract your chest and triceps. Straighten your arms, returning to starting position. Do not lock your elbows.

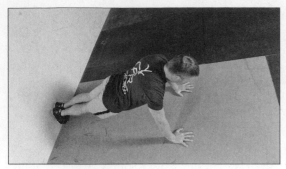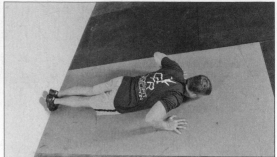

Full pushup.

Pushups can become infinitely harder, and many variations can be performed. If 20 standard pushups become easy for you, start elevating your feet. The higher you elevate your feet, the harder the pushup will become. You can also change your hand positions—under your shoulders, wider than your shoulders, in front of your shoulders, or touching.

Lunges

The lunge is a weight-training exercise that's used to strengthen the quadriceps muscles, the gluteal muscles, and the muscles comprising the hamstrings. A long lunge emphasizes the glutes, whereas a short lunge emphasizes the quadriceps.

1. Stand straight, looking forward, with your legs hip distance apart. Pretend that you have a clock lying on the ground in front of you, with 12:00 being directly ahead.

2. Step one leg forward; if you move your left leg first, it would land on 11:00; if you move your right leg first, it would land on 1:00. Land on your heel and roll your foot down flat against the floor. You should get far enough forward that you keep the shin of your front leg vertical but don't let your toe go over your knee. It's very important to make sure your foot, ankle, and knee stay in alignment. Many people experience knee pain when performing lunges because the knee goes over the ankle and foot and stresses their patella tendon.

3. Step your rear leg forward and then alternate legs with each step. This is essentially just an exaggerated walking step. It's common to have one leg that's more stable than the other. With continuing work on lunges, you'll strengthen the weaker leg.

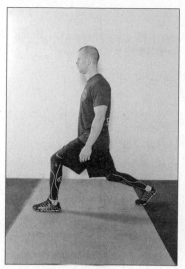 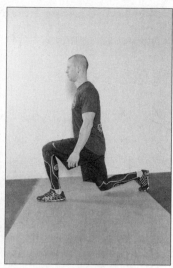

Lunge.

Intermediate: Weighted Walking Lunge

For the weighted walking lunge, hold the dumbbells at your sides and keep looking straight ahead. Remember to hold your core still and keep your knee tracking with your toe. Don't let your knee go over your toe.

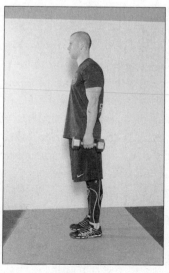 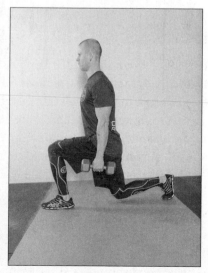

Weighted walking lunge.

Advanced: Overhead Walking Lunge

For the overhead walking lunge, hold your core still and hold the dumbbells over your head. Remember to keep looking straight ahead and keep your knee tracking over your toe.

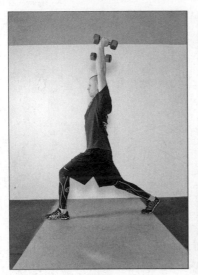 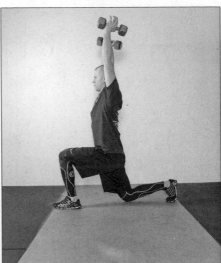

Overhead walking lunge.

Dead Lift

The dead lift, though incredibly simple, has a significant ability to increase strength from head to toe. It's one of the most functional moves you have, and it's critical whether you want to increase your metabolism, decrease body fat, increase strength, increase lean muscle mass, rehabilitate your back, improve athletic performance, or maintain independence as a senior. In reality, it's no more than taking something up off the ground. You do it many times every day as you go about your daily tasks: a bag of dog food, the trash, a suitcase, your toddler, and so on.

Here's how you do the dead lift:

1. Stand with your feet under your hips. Grip the dumbbells or bar, keeping your arms straight.

2. Have your shoulders slightly forward of the bar and the inside of the elbows facing one another. Keep your chest up and inflated and your abdominal muscles tight.

3. Keep your arms locked and not pulling up. Keep your shoulders back and down. Keep your weight on your heels, and with your abdominal muscles tight and your back straight, stand so that the bar or dumbbells stay close to your legs and essentially travel straight up and down.

4. Keep looking straight ahead. Stand straight up, keeping your back flat and your arms locked.

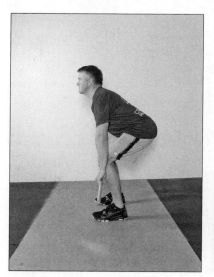 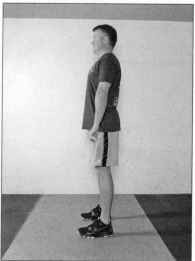

Dead lift.

Beginner: Suitcase Dead Lift

Suitcase dead lifting is done with one dumbbell. The dumbbell suitcase dead lift is initiated by placing the dumbbell to one side. The feet are spaced evenly about shoulder width apart.

Grasp the dumbbell, tighten the core, and lift while pressing through the heels and maintaining a firm and fixed flat back position. Make sure your hand is straight and doing nothing more than holding on to the load, not bending at the elbow or shrugging from the shoulder.

Not everyone has the mobility to squat this deep. If you cannot assume a correct starting position, with eyes forward, chest up, and back flat, then the barbells should be elevated.

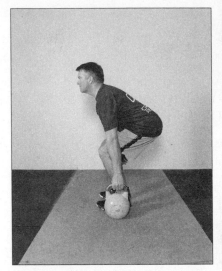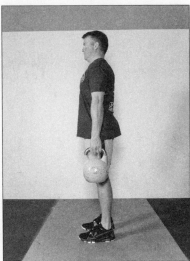

Suitcase dead lift.

Intermediate: Dumbbell Standard Dead Lift

See the previous description; however, use one dumbbell in each hand.

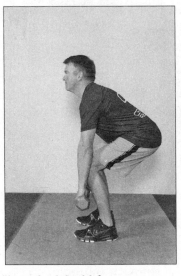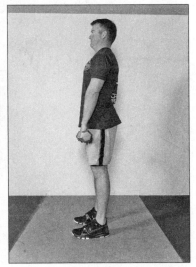

Dumbbell standard dead lift.

Advanced: Single-Leg Dead Lift

Performing a single-leg dead lift allows you to target the muscles one leg at a time. It's more challenging than a regular dead lift and requires more balance and agility.

1. Stand holding weights in front of your thighs and place your left leg out behind you with the toe lightly touching the floor (or lift it completely off the floor for more of a challenge). Use light weights until you get the hang of it.

2. Keeping the shoulders back, abs in, and back straight, tip from the hips and lower the weight toward the floor. Don't round your shoulders forward.

3. Lower as far as your flexibility allows. You can bend the knee slightly if you need to. This is not a squat, but a move that comes from the hips. Keep your knee at the same angle throughout the movement.

4. Push into the heel to go back to starting position.

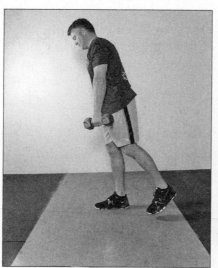 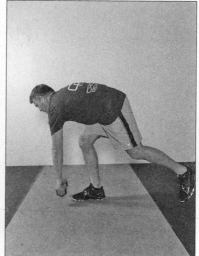

Single-leg dead lift.

Burpee

The burpee is a full-body exercise used in strength training as an aerobic exercise. It's performed in five steps. There are no different levels to a burpee. Essentially, you're lying all the way down on the ground, standing all the way up, and jumping in place. It doesn't get more functional than that!

1. Begin in a standing position.

2. Drop into a squat position with your hands on the ground.

3. Kick your feet back while lowering yourself into a pushup.

4. Pull your feet back to your hands and start to stand up.

5. Leap up as high as possible from the squat position with your arms overhead (you may also clap your hands above your head at the peak of your jump).

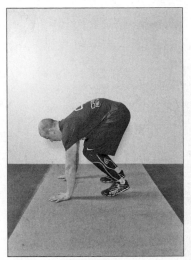 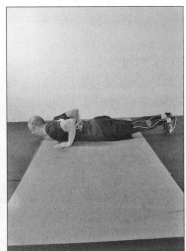 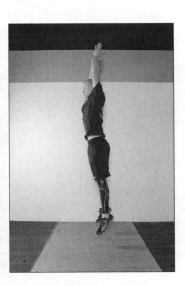

Burpee.

Variations of burpees that are more challenging include:

- Long-jump burpee: The athlete jumps forward, not upward.

- Tuck-jump burpee: The athlete pulls his knees to his chest (tucks) at the peak of the jump.

- Jump-over burpee: The athlete jumps over an obstacle between burpees.

- Box-jump burpee: The athlete jumps onto a box, rather than straight up and down.

Kettle Bell Swing (or Dumbbell Swing)

The swing is an excellent movement to help build your core, including your legs, butt, back, and abdominal muscles. This really allows you to work out your entire body at once. As you get better, you can move from bringing the dumbbell just to a level out in front of you (Russian swing) to eventually bringing it up over your head (American swing). By pushing your bottom back and bringing your hips forward, you can generate much more power to propel the dumbbell or kettle bell higher.

Beginner: Russian Swing

Start with a very light dumbbell/kettle bell.

1. Hold the handle with both hands. Keep your abdominal muscles tight and stand tall. Keep your weight in your heels and your feet about shoulder width apart.

2. Push your butt back and allow the dumbbell/kettle bell to swing back slightly.

3. Thrust your hips forward and tighten your butt. This will allow the dumbbell/ kettle bell to swing up to the level of your navel or chest. Remember, your arms are just there to guide the dumbbell/kettle bell; they should not be doing the work. Your butt and hamstrings should be.

4. "Catch" the dumbbell/kettle bell as it falls. Using the momentum you're creating, move your hips forward again to swing the dumbbell/kettle bell forward again. Correctly done, this movement should be felt in your butt and hamstrings, not your back.

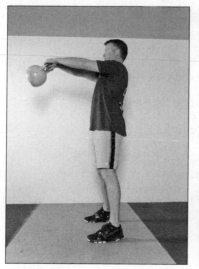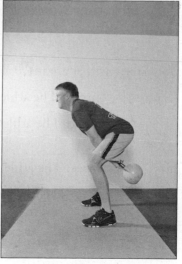

Russian swing.

Intermediate: Single Hand Swing

The technique for one-handed swings is identical to the two-handed variety except obviously you hold the kettle bell with one hand only.

1. Place the kettle bell between your feet and bend your knees to get into the starting position.

2. Grip the kettle bell tightly, look forward, and keep your back flat. Swing the kettle bell up from between your legs forcefully.

3. At the top, let gravity slow the kettle bell down before letting it swing back down between your legs. As it gets to the bottom, contract your glutes and hamstrings to catch it, and then as quickly as possible, reverse the direction and explode back up again.

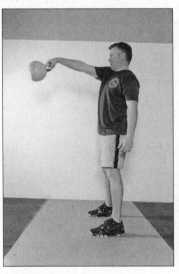 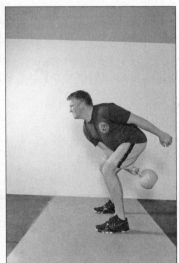

Single hand swing.

Advanced: American Swing

This is the same basic movement as the beginner swing. However, this time the apex or top of the arc of the dumbbell/kettle bell will be over your head. Make sure to keep your core muscles very tight as you swing it over your head. Use the momentum from each downward swing to help propel the dumbbell/kettle bell back up again.

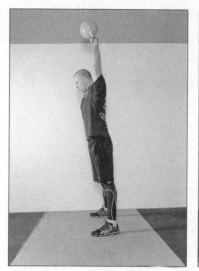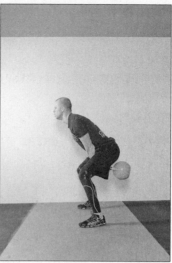

American swing.

Interval Exercises

Interval workouts alternate high-intensity effort with lower-intensity effort. The benefit of this type of workout is that your metabolism increases and you continue to burn calories long after you stop working out. I talked earlier about the fact that if you closely watch children at play, many other games (tag, kickball, baseball, etc.) are actually done in intervals. Many sports are also done in start and stop motions, with periods of sprinting followed by jogging or rest. Keep in mind that many of the intervals are actually anaerobic training. Sports like baseball, football, gymnastics, soccer, volleyball, wrestling, and weight lifting are all intervals that require the majority of training time spent in anaerobic activity.

There are a number of ways to set up your own interval workouts. These are discussed in the following sections.

Standard Interval Workouts

The standard interval workout is used with any activity or combination of activities and includes the following.

- 5 minutes warm-up (lighter intensity)
- 1 minute of moderate- to high-intensity work followed by 30 seconds of low-intensity work (repeat 6–10 times)
- 3–5 minutes cool down (lighter intensity)

Pyramid Interval Workouts

Pyramid interval workouts can be used with any activity or combination of activities. They involve the following:

- 5 minutes warm-up
- 30 seconds high intensity
- 30 seconds low intensity

Repeat high intensity and low intensity for 45 seconds and 60 seconds, and then do 90 seconds of high intensity. After 90 seconds, do 60 seconds of high intensity and 60 seconds of low intensity, and then repeat this for 45 seconds and 30 seconds. Finally, cool down for 3 to 5 minutes.

Tabata Exercises

Dr. Tabata, of the National Institute of Fitness and Sports in Japan, found that high-intensity, intermittent training improved both anaerobic and aerobic energy supply systems significantly. His exercises consist of intermittent training using eight sets of 20 seconds at maximum intensity with 10 seconds of rest between each bout. The beauty of these is that, within four minutes, you get an incredibly intense workout. I often do them with squats, sit-ups, or pushups. However, you could get creative and do them with almost anything: sprinting, rowing, cycling, pull-ups, jump rope, and so on.

Tabata Intervals

These intervals can be done with pushups, squats, sit-ups, pull-ups, sprints, rowing, cycling, and so on. Use the following for timing in between exercises:

- 20 seconds maximum effort
- 10 seconds rest
- Repeat eight times for a total of 4 minutes work and rest

You can keep track of how you do by counting the number of reps you get in each 20-second bout and taking the lowest number of all 8 bouts as your score. For example, if you're doing Tabata squats and can do 15 squats in the first bout, 16 in the second, 14 in the third, 15 in the fourth, 13 in the fifth, 12 in the sixth, 14 in the seventh, and 13 in the eighth, your score would be 12 because that was your lowest number of reps.

Sample Workouts

Each of these workouts can be made harder by increasing the difficulty of the movements. As you're learning the workouts, start with the beginner movements and, as you increase your strength, move to intermediate and advanced movements. You can also increase the time allotted for some of the As Many Rounds As Possible (AMRAP) workouts.

Note the basic patterns of the workouts, and as you gain more experience, feel free to mix them up a little bit. For example, for workout #1, you may want to add sit-ups or increase the number of reps to 15 per exercise. The goal is to get variety and maintain the intervals with higher intensity and lower intensity. Make sure you keep track of your time or the number of rounds you complete for each given group of exercises. (I would like to thank Andrew Romeo at CrossFit Revelation [www.CrossFitRevelation.com] for designing these workouts for me.)

Workout #1: Set a timer for 12 minutes, and perform AMRAP of the following three exercises: 15 squats, 10 pushups, and 5 burpees.

If you're not challenged by 12 minutes, increase your workout time to 20 minutes. This variation will help you mix up your workout: Jump rope for 30 reps, do 10 sit-ups, and do 5 burpees.

The following is another variation: Sprint 100 m/row 100 m/bike 100 m (easiest on stationary equipment), do 15 squats, and do 5 burpees.

Workout #2: Perform three rounds as fast as possible. Form comes first; do not sacrifice your form and technique to go more quickly.

- 20 dead lifts
- 20 pushups
- 20 kettle bell swings

Workout #3: In the first minute, perform five burpees. For the remainder of the minute, complete as many squats as possible. When you get to the next minute, perform five more burpees and complete the minute with squats. Continue the workout until you have completed 100 squats. Mark down the time it took you to complete 100 squats while doing five burpees at the beginning of each minute.

Workout #4: Complete AMRAP in 10 minutes. As you get more proficient, move to 15 minutes, and then 20 minutes.

- 10 lunges (5 per leg)
- 10 kettle bell swings
- 10 pushups

Workout #5: Complete four rounds for time: Run 400 m (¼ mile) and do 50 squats.

Workout #6: Complete 10 rounds for time. Make sure you focus on your form for the dead lifts. Do 5 dead lifts, 5 lunges, and 5 burpees.

Exercises for Travel

The beauty of these intervals and workouts is that many of them can be done anywhere, and they don't take a long time. For instance, when traveling, I can pack a jump rope and my workout clothes and get a workout in even if the hotel doesn't have an exercise facility. The Tabata exercises can be done in your room, and so can workout #1 and workout #3. If you have a gym facility available, you can use the treadmill, stationary bicycle, or rowing machines to do Tabata exercises or spice up some of the other workouts. If you can run outside, workout #5 can be done anywhere. If you're in a high-rise hotel, sprint up and down the stairs. Get creative! The bottom line is that you have no excuse not to be able to get a workout in, even if you travel.

The Least You Need to Know

- You need to use both aerobic and anaerobic pathways to get your energy level where it needs to be when you do any kind of exercise.
- Interval training takes less time than traditional training, and because you work at a much higher intensity, it helps with aerobic and anaerobic capacity.
- Dumbbells can add variety and intensity to your exercises.
- You can do a number of workouts with no equipment; you can always work out, even while traveling.

Evaluate Your Eating Habits

In This Chapter

- Maintaining your enthusiasm
- Overcoming stress eating
- Listening to your body
- Drinking water to control hunger

In this chapter, I discuss four important eating habits—listening to your body's cues, emotional eating, stress eating, and adequate hydration. Evaluate the role these habits play in the way you eat and your daily food intake. Based on what you learn, you may want to develop some new, more positive habits to replace those that are sabotaging your diet.

Maintaining Your Enthusiasm

It's amazing to think of the power your body has over your emotions. In their book *The Astonishing Power of Emotions*, Esther and Jerry Hicks discuss how the way you feel about your actions affects you. Creating a healthy body that you feel good about is not as much about making things happen through action as it is about allowing the things you desire to happen.

The way you allow things to happen is by aligning how you feel with what you want. For example, if you think back on the times in your life when you tried to diet, you'll probably find examples in which action made a difference, such as reducing food consumption or increasing exercise to lose weight. However, you probably can think of times when your thoughts and emotions were not aligned with your goal, and you "fell off the wagon."

The enthusiasm you feel when you first start a new weight-loss program is an important emotion. That positive emotion is what gives you the power to follow through on your actions of healthy eating, stress management, and exercise. As you imagine your fit, healthy body, you're creating it and moving yourself closer to it. However, if, when you see yourself in the mirror, the changes aren't happening fast enough and you judge yourself harshly, your old patterns and beliefs cause discord, and you move yourself away from your ideal body. The best way to bring your body to a new place is to see it differently from the way it was. In the words of Esther and Jerry, "You cannot create a new reality while looking at your current reality."

You have no choice but to be in the body you're in right now. What you can change is how you view your body and whether you choose to make yourself feel a little better or a little worse. Those choices make all the difference because, in the long run, they are what will move you closer to your ideal body.

It's not the action that matters; it's how you're feeling about what you're doing. If you focus on feeling enthusiasm rather than discouragement, you'll start finding more and more options and actions that keep you feeling better. As you move with the new ideas and options rather than struggle against them, things will be easier. At the end of the day, if your only choices are to make things easier or make them harder, why would you ever choose harder? Yet people do that all the time. They create struggles with themselves and irritation rather than finding benefits and enthusiasm in their undertakings.

As you see improvements in your body, you'll see an increase in your feeling of enthusiasm. Hold on to that feeling and have gratitude for it. That's the source of power you should use to move toward your ideal body. As you achieve your fit, healthy body, you may note that this time it wasn't as difficult to lose weight and feel healthier. This time, you did it with minimal struggle.

Some statements to help you maintain your enthusiasm are as follows:

- It's good to have choices about what I eat.

- I know that I am eating in a way that will balance my hormones.

- I have many options for my meals.

- I get to eat five times a day!

- I like taking care of myself!

Stop Eating in Response to Stress

When you're in a situation in which you have significant stress or you're at your weakest point emotionally, you can have the strongest cravings for food. You may choose food for comfort, to help you with a difficult problem, to alleviate your stress, or to keep you from being bored. You may not even be aware that you do these things. Your body usually craves sweets during these times because the cortisol triggered by stress will raise the blood sugar. As the blood sugar rises in response to cortisol, insulin acts to push the sugar from the blood into the cells. If insulin does its job "too well," your blood sugar drops and your body starts craving sugars and sweets to bring it back up again.

THAT'S QUOTABLE

"We are all dietetic sinners; only a small percent of what we eat nourishes us; the balance goes to waste and loss of energy."

—William Osler

Stress eating can wreak havoc on weight-loss efforts. Usually, when you're stressed out, you don't go running for the carrots and celery. You crave high-calorie, refined-carbohydrate, processed, full-of-trans-fats foods—and you tend to eat a whole lot of them! Stress eating is eating as a way to suppress or soothe negative emotions, such as anxiety, anger, fear, boredom, sadness, and loneliness. Both major life events and the hassles of daily life can trigger negative emotions that lead to stress eating and disrupt your weight-loss efforts. Here are some of the triggers for stress and emotional eating:

- A major loss
- Anxiety or depression
- Bad weather
- Boredom
- Fatigue
- Financial pressures
- Health problems
- Job problems, work stress, or unemployment
- Moving
- Relationship conflicts

Although some people actually eat less in the face of strong emotions, if you're in emotional distress, you may turn to impulsive or binge eating—you may rapidly eat whatever's convenient, without even enjoying it. In fact, your emotions may become so tied to your eating habits that you automatically reach for a sweet treat whenever you're angry or stressed without stopping to think about what you're doing.

Food also serves as a distraction. If you're worried about an upcoming event or stewing over a conflict, for instance, you may focus on eating comfort food instead of dealing with the painful situation. Whatever emotions drive you to overeat, the end result is often the same. The emotions return, and you may also now bear the burden of guilt about setting back your weight-loss goal.

There's good news! Although negative emotions can trigger emotional eating, you can take steps to regain control of your eating habits and get back to a healthy lifestyle.

Here are tips to reduce stress eating:

- **Tame your stress.** If stress contributes to your emotional eating, try a stress management technique, such as yoga, meditation, or relaxation.

- **Check to see whether you're really hungry.** Is your hunger physical or emotional? If you ate just a few hours ago and don't have a rumbling stomach, you're probably not really hungry. Give the craving a little time to pass.

- **Keep a food diary.** Write down what you eat, how much you eat, when you eat, how you're feeling when you eat, and how hungry you are. Over time, you may see patterns emerge that reveal the connection between mood and food.

- **Get support.** Remember Principle #7? You're more likely to give in to emotional eating if you lack a good support network. Lean on family and friends or consider joining a support group.

- **Fight boredom.** Instead of snacking when you're not truly hungry, distract yourself. Take a walk, watch a movie, play with your cat, listen to music, read, or call a friend and catch up.

- **Remove temptation.** Don't keep supplies of comfort foods in your home if they're hard for you to resist. And if you feel angry or blue, postpone your trip to the grocery store until you're sure that you have your emotions in check.

- **Don't deprive yourself.** When you're trying to achieve a weight-loss goal, you may limit your calories too much, eat the same foods frequently, and banish the treats you enjoy. This may just serve to increase your food cravings, especially in response to emotions. Let yourself enjoy an occasional treat and get plenty of variety to help curb cravings.

> **TRUSTY TIP**
>
> If you feel the urge to eat between meals, choose a balanced snack including protein, fruit/veggies, and healthy fats. You could try veggies and hummus, apples and almond butter, grilled chicken salad, deviled eggs, or almonds.

- **Get enough sleep.** If you're constantly tired, you might snack to try to give yourself an energy boost. Take a nap or go to bed earlier instead.

- **Seek therapy.** If you've tried self-help options but you still can't get control of your emotional eating, consider therapy with a professional mental health provider. Therapy can help you understand the motivations behind your emotional eating and help you learn new coping skills. Therapy can also help you discover whether you may have an eating disorder, which is sometimes connected to emotional eating.

Listen to Your Body's Cues

Your appetite control mechanism maintains a delicate balance between the energy you require and the food you take in. The communication occurs between hormones from your endocrine system and neurotransmitters from your brain. Normally, when your stomach is empty, it secretes hormones to let your brain know. Your brain triggers the hunger response to encourage you to look for food and prepares your stomach as well. After you eat, the food enters your stomach and intestines and causes the secretion of more hormones to help with digestion. When your stomach is full, your stomach and your fat cells send messages to your brain to let you know that you're full. Then you should stop eating, your liver and intestines should continue digestion, and you should either burn or store your sugar and fat.

By overriding your appetite cues, you create an imbalance between the molecules that control hunger within in your body. You end up having an appetite that can't be satisfied; you're hungry right after you finish eating. Your body might store fat when it should be burning it or the other way around. This leads to a damaged metabolism and weight gain.

Tips for regaining control of your appetite include:

- Don't eat processed food that contains high fructose corn syrup, refined carbohydrates, or trans fats.

- Focus on fiber, which helps slow down the absorption of sugar. This reduces your appetite, and you'll stay full longer. Remember, fresh fruits and vegetables have a great deal of fiber.

- Don't use artificial sweeteners. One of the side effects of sweeteners is a stimulation of hunger due to miscommunication between your brain and your insulin response.

- Eat regularly throughout the day and at about the same time each day. People who eat regularly timed meals and snacks have a reduction in their overall food intake throughout the course of the day.

Differentiate Hunger from Thirst

Water makes up 55 to 60 percent of your body. Only oxygen is more critical than water, and it is necessary for every reaction in your body. Water is also important for detoxification. Therefore, the lower the water content in your body, the less likely you'll be to adequately detoxify. Remember, toxins are stored in fat, and the more toxins you have, the more fat you hang on to, and the less weight you're able to lose.

Do you ever notice that even after eating a good-sized meal you're still hungry? Well, believe it or not, the hunger that you're feeling could be a sign of dehydration. For 37 percent of Americans, the thirst mechanism is so weak that it's often mistaken for hunger. Therefore, many people misinterpret dehydration as hunger, which is an easy mistake to make. It's definitely worth the effort to drink a glass of water and wait a few minutes if you're not sure that you're truly hungry, especially at night. One glass of water shut down midnight hunger pangs for almost 100 percent of the dieters in a University of Washington study.

TRUSTY TIP

If you're hungry shortly after eating, check to see how much water you've had so far that day. You may not need food, but you do need water.

Water is the best beverage for managing dehydration. Beverages such as sodas, iced teas, and coffee are dehydrating agents because of the sugar and caffeine content. Of note, caffeinated coffee and iced tea are only mildly dehydrating. However, it's a good idea to monitor your intake of these drinks, as the caffeine doses are addictive and may create stress for your adrenals.

A guideline for daily water intake is to take your weight and divide by 2. The answer is the amount of water you should drink daily in ounces. For instance, someone who weighs 150 pounds should drink 75 ounces of water per day. Another good indicator that you are getting enough water is that your urine should be pale yellow with the exception of your first urine each morning.

Because water is so important, you have many cues to make sure you take in enough. One obvious cue is thirst. In truth, thirst will not keep you ideally hydrated. Thirst is not a fuel gauge; it's a warning light. It begins after you're already mildly dehydrated, doesn't increase in intensity proportionately with your degree of dehydration, and is relieved before you're fully rehydrated. The amount of water loss that occurs before symptoms of dehydration set in varies from person to person. However, it is thought that 75 percent of Americans are chronically dehydrated.

You can normally drink water equal to about 1 percent of your body weight without causing excessive, inconvenient urination. One or 2 pints of water early in the day can give you a head start on avoiding thirst (and dehydration—remember, thirst means you're already dehydrated).

Because thirst begins at 2 percent dehydration, it begins after a loss of 2 percent of your usual body weight. You're not conscious of the first 1 percent that you're always short of, and after you're thirsty, you can get back to your mildly parched and normal state by drinking water equal to 1 percent of your body weight.

The delay of thirst is actually useful: if you became thirsty as soon as you need an ounce of water, you'd be continually looking for water, which is a waste of time. If thirst was exactly proportional to the need, you'd be in agonies of thirst. Thirst is a reliable signal that you need to drink a pint to a quart of water (depending on your size) right now and to, in general, increase how much fluid you consume and how often.

TRUSTY TIP

If any of these signs occur, you may be dehydrated: hunger, pain (lower back), cramps, dizziness, fatigue, headache, and constipation.

The Least You Need to Know

- You can regain control of your appetite by eating whole foods and eliminating trans fats, refined carbohydrates, and high fructose corn syrup.

- The emotion with which you undertake weight loss is more important than the actions themselves.

- By focusing on eating healthier foods and reducing stress, you can break the cycle of stress eating and hormone imbalance.

- By the time you're thirsty, you have lost 2 to 3 percent of your body weight in water, and you're dehydrated, which can lead to fatigue, reduced metabolism, and a decreased ability to detoxify.

- The lower the water content in your body, the less likely you'll be to adequately detoxify.

Establish a
Support Network

In This Chapter

- Enlisting help to be accountable to your goals
- Face-to-face and online support groups
- How to break the ice with a potential diet buddy

You've heard the saying, "Two heads are better than one." When trying to lose weight, enlisting a partner or group to be your cheerleaders and remind you to eat right and exercise can make the difference between success and failure. From identifying the best weight-loss buddy for you to learning how to break the ice with a potential diet buddy, this chapter gives tips on how to enlist help in your quest for losing weight.

Choosing a Weight-Loss Buddy

Start the process for identifying a buddy by making a list of potential candidates. Make sure you know the personalities of those people you are considering; you want to set yourself up to succeed by working with someone with whom you communicate well. It is important that you "click." Only you know whether you want someone who is a cheerleader, an easygoing companion, or a bossy type to move you toward your health and weight-loss goals.

If you don't know anyone who is trying to lose weight, no rule says you can't pick a nondieter to be your weight-loss buddy. She might have lost weight previously and know all too well how hard it is to stay focused on a diet. Or she might be an empathetic friend who is willing to be a partner and sounding board. The nice thing about having a nondieter as your buddy is that your whole relationship is not based on losing weight. You can do things with your friend that are for her and are not necessarily weight-loss related.

One of the best things a weight-loss buddy can do for you is hold you accountable for your eating habits and lifestyle changes. You and your buddy can agree to reinforce positive behavior and offer each other a lot of praise. It takes 21 days to make a habit, and if your new behaviors are not reinforced, it'll be all that much harder to last for that long.

It's important to make sure that your weight-loss buddy has your best interests at heart. If you're both on a diet, there might be weeks during which one of you loses weight and the other one doesn't. Those are the weeks when you'll both need to strive to support each other. Having a buddy available to share in your disappointments will make it easier to handle. You'll be less likely to get discouraged and more able to maintain your enthusiasm.

Weight loss might be more effective with a buddy who exercises at the same intensity that you do. If one is significantly faster than the other, someone is going to have to change their pace. This can create stress.

The buddy system works best if you can see each other in person. If there are no other options, a long-distance buddy is certainly better than no support at all.

If you can't find a suitable weight-loss buddy in your circle of friends and acquaintances, look online or in your community. You can post an invitation for a weight-loss buddy at your church, work, social group, and at a local weight-loss meeting such as Weight Watchers. It's all about community.

Stop Hiding: Tips and Tricks

Many people find it difficult to ask for help. Interestingly, you might have absolutely no problem helping those around you, sometimes to the point at which their needs come before yours. One of the first things you need to believe before you can ask for help is that you are valuable and deserve it.

I often ask my patients who think they might be a burden to others to imagine the scenario in reverse. What if you had a family member who, in order to significantly improve their health, needed to lose weight? What if that family member felt comfortable with you and asked for your support as she tried to lose weight? If you had the ability to do it, would you help her?

Most of my patients would definitely help their family members. They wouldn't think twice! But for some reason, they don't think the same would apply to them. The reality is, if they would be willing to help somebody else, there should be no reason that others should not be willing to do it for them as well.

Vulnerability is not a weakness; it's actually a sign of strength because you're willing to show others your human side. That is often something people can relate to, and the fact that they can find something in common with you might even increase their respect for you. Asking for help tells others that, even if you don't have all the answers, you're willing to look for them.

Many people think that holding things in or keeping their personal issues secret makes them stronger or secure. Although I don't recommend "spilling your guts" to everyone out on the street, by not letting anyone really "know" you, including your questions and your issues, you keep yourself socially isolated. Just like realizing that vulnerability is not a weakness, seeking counsel from others connects you with them as well. At the same time, you can realize that you're not alone with your problems and concerns. That can help reduce stress and keep your cortisol level down, which, of course, is paramount in your weight-loss efforts.

I talked about the caregiver role and self-sacrifice in Chapter 10. Thinking that you can't ask for help because it will bother others is a form of self-sacrifice that can end up creating significant problems for you. Doing and being it all can really do you in. If you're too self-sufficient, you can create stress levels and increased cortisol demands that lead to hormone imbalance and further weight gain. Some of my patients say to me, "I love to give, and I hate when others help me." I laugh and tell them that they're setting themselves up for disaster. With practice, you can learn to be comfortable when others help you.

If you look at highly successful people, the ones who are healthy know how to ask for help. They will tell you that one of the biggest keys to success is knowing your strengths and weaknesses. No one is perfect; we all have strengths and weaknesses. The healthy people know how to delegate. They know how to ask for help and how to trust the talents of those around them. They create a team of people whom they can rely on to help them find answers and pick up the slack when necessary to reach their overall goals. You can do the same thing to reach your weight-loss goals.

You can break the ice with someone and ask for help in several ways. If you're really nervous, you can even ask what he would suggest for a "friend" of yours. Listen to his answer and, if you're comfortable, tell him the truth is that the "friend" is actually you! It's a good way to start a conversation if you're really stuck. However, don't do this too often. The best thing to do is just believe that you're worthy of someone's help and support.

Following are some "ice breakers" you can use to ask for help:

- I need to lose weight to improve my health. Could you help me?

- Could you do me a favor and help me avoid my weight-loss "danger zones" like buffets?

- I need to start exercising. Would you join a class with me so I don't have to go alone?

- Can you help me find activities that don't center on food?

- I noticed how good you look with your weight loss. Would you be willing to help me with mine?

- I was thinking of learning how to meditate to relieve stress. Do you have any suggestions?

How to Pick a Support Group

A support system can be a source of strength as you go through the ups and downs of changing your eating habits and your lifestyle. One of the first things to do is decide what will work best for you. Do you want an Internet support forum and the availability to chat anonymously with anyone 24/7? You can also consider a face-to-face support group, such as Overeaters Anonymous. Either way, you can talk with people who have the same problems you have. You can both give and get advice.

Many face-to-face support groups allow members to weigh themselves, discuss their challenges, offer advice, celebrate each other's success, and exchange recipes. A study by the National Weight Control Registry showed that people who've lost weight and continued support group meetings every other week for a year were able to maintain their weight loss. Those that didn't continue with support regained almost half of the weight they lost.

We've talked about this before, but it bears repeating: the reason that both online and face-to-face support groups work is accountability. At each meeting, you have to share with the other dieters what you ate, what lifestyle changes you're making, how much you're exercising, and how much weight you've lost. If you have to report these things, you're more likely to make sure you're doing them. This also contributes to the amount of control you have regarding your ability to lose weight. In a group setting, not only are you motivated by others, but you might motivate them by showing them your successes.

Here are some of the top face-to-face weight-loss support groups to consider:

- TOPS (Take Off Pounds Sensibly)
- Weight Watchers
- Jenny Craig
- University medical centers: Check in your local area
- Hospitals: Check in your local area
- Church groups: Check in your local area
- Overeaters Anonymous

Online Support Groups

More and more dieters are turning to the Internet to find help losing weight. For one thing, it's convenient and time saving, especially if you don't live near a weight-loss center. Also, given the time constraints of work and family, commitments can get in the way of going to meetings, and the Internet may be a better option for you. Internet groups are often more economical than face-to-face groups. And participants save on gas and travel time.

Message boards are important features of Internet groups. You'll not only find moral support and encouragement, but helpful suggestions and tips. You can share recipes and meal plans. When you feel stuck in a rut, you can learn what helps others stay focused on their food plans. Find someone else who's dieting, whether it's on a message board or someone you know personally, to share your successes as well as setbacks. By being accountable, you're more likely to stay on your program and reach your goal. Finally, realize that online dieting works for many, but not everyone. If you find it's not working for you, then explore other options. Don't give up!

Online diet program options include:

- **eDiets (www.ediets.com)**—eDiets encompasses all the other online diet programs. Besides offering convenience, eDiets endorses a number of commercial diet programs, as well as offering plans tailored for dieters with special medical needs.

- **Weight Watchers Online (www.weightwatchers.com)**—Weight Watchers Online is another good, affordable program. It's packed with helpful tips, menus, and recipes. Weight Watchers Online also provides a weight tracker, community message boards, and helpful tools.

- **The South Beach Diet Online (www.southbeachdiet.com)**—Similar to Weight Watchers Online, the South Beach Diet Online also offers a weight tracker, as well as message boards, food guide, a personal online journal, and other extras.

- **Jenny Craig Online Dieting (http://jennycraig.com)**—Jenny Craig's at-home weight-loss program affords the same benefits as those who go to local Jenny Craig centers. You'll receive one-on-one weekly phone support during which a trained counselor helps you plan your weekly menus and activities.

- **Weight Loss Buddy (www.weightlossbuddy.com)**—This is a free program but offers a profile page, a team page, free diet planning, and a number of blogs by their extensive list of experts.

- **SparkPeople (www.sparkpeople.com)**—SparkPeople's mission is to *spark* millions of *people* to live healthier lives and reach their goals. They offer personalized diet plans, fitness plans, a calorie counter, a workout tracker, exercise videos, answers from dietitians and trainers on personal message boards, and connection to other people.

The Least You Need to Know

- Choose a weight-loss buddy whose personality traits you're most likely to respond to.
- Sharing your disappointments with someone else who can relate might help you maintain your enthusiasm.
- Research shows that dieters who lose weight and continue with a support group for the following year maintain their weight loss.
- Vulnerability is not a weakness.
- Support groups work whether they are face-to-face or online.

Continuing Success

This part gives you the framework to design your personal action plan for hormone balance and weight loss, with information specifically tailored to children, teens, men, women, and seniors. The action plan is supplemented with worksheets that allow you to track your daily progress. In addition, you will track your exercise results and measurements, which will allow you to clearly see your progress.

I provide a large number of meal suggestions and food tables listing the different foods that are allowed in a format that lets you mix and match the foods to your own tastes. There are also 28-day menu plans for Phase I and Phase II of the diet with a number of amazing recipes.

Once you complete Phase I, Phase II gives you the framework to continue eating for optimal health. I also discuss symptoms of food sensitivity so you can determine whether or not grains or dairy will affect your future weight loss.

Finally, this part ends with the part of the plan where you start to make it work especially for you. You'll use action plan worksheets to help you track your eating, stress management, and exercising efforts.

Phase I: 30-Day Action Plan

In This Chapter

- Introducing Phase I
- Foods for Phase I
- Meal plans
- Recipes for your hormone weight-loss plan

You are on Phase I for the first 30 days of the hormone weight-loss diet, although you can stay on it for a longer period of time if you have more weight or sizes to lose. When you begin this plan, you might be concerned about all of the changes you are making in your diet and what they mean for your taste buds, but the truth is that this phase actually includes an unlimited number of food combinations so that, once you get the hang of it, you will not be bored.

This chapter gives you the information you need to get started on the diet, including meal plans and recipes.

Phase I of the Hormone Weight-Loss Diet

During Phase I, remove all grains and dairy products from your diet. This is to help your body reduce inflammation and irritation, which reduces cortisol demand and makes it easier for you to lose weight. This phase also helps you detoxify your system.

When you move on to Phase II, you can add a few servings of full-fat dairy and gluten-free whole grains back into your diet. If you notice that you're gaining weight again, remove them from your diet until your metabolism is more stable.

Counting calories is in the past. Because you're eating simple, clean food, you will naturally start to eat what your body needs and feel satisfied. Remember to include protein, fats, and vegetables with each meal.

If you only need to lose one size, you can include two servings of fruit per day. If you need to lose two sizes or more, limit your fruit serving to one per day and make sure you're eating only low glycemic index fruits.

Get Your Kitchen Ready

One of the key things to do as you get ready for Phase I is to get rid of everything in your kitchen that might wreak havoc with your diet. If you don't have forbidden products in your kitchen, you won't be tempted to eat them in a moment of weakness. Your family might not be happy with you at first, but hopefully they will follow your example and eliminate all unhealthy foods from their diets.

Make sure you remove everything that contains hydrogenated or partially hydrogenated fats, refined carbohydrates like white flour and white sugar, and high fructose corn syrup. In addition, get rid of and don't purchase tomato products in cans; buy them in glass bottles.

Try to buy organic food that is antibiotic and hormone free as often as possible. A number of food chains such as Whole Foods, Wild Oats, and Trader Joe's make purchasing organic foods easier. And most grocery chains now carry their own lines of organic foods. Also, make sure that you're drinking clean, filtered water.

Phase I Food Table

I've included a table of foods that are allowed during Phase I of this diet. As a general rule, choose a protein source and add some vegetables, healthy fats, and spices. You can cook them in a variety of ways, including baking, broiling, grilling, and stir-frying.

Animal Proteins (including eggs, meat, and seafood)	Other Proteins (beans, nuts, and legumes)	Starchy Vegetables (acceptable, but eat fewer and combine with fats and proteins)	Nonstarchy Vegetables (eat in unlimited quantities and at every meal and for snacks)	Fruits (LG = Low Glycemic Index; MG = Medium Glycemic Index; HG = High Glycemic Index)	Fats	Grains and Flours (available for Phase II)	Miscellaneous Items
Eggs	Black beans	Beets	Artichokes	Blackberries (LG)	Almond oil	Quinoa	Vinegars
Beef (organic, grass-fed)	Black-eyed peas	Carrots (cooked)	Arugula	Blueberries (LG)	Avocado oil	Whole-grain brown rice	Lemon juice and zest
Bison	Garbanzo beans	Jerusalem artichoke	Asparagus	Boysenberries (LG)	Butter	Amaranth	Dried and fresh herbs
Chicken	Kidney beans	Parsnips	Beet top	Grapefruit (LG)	Canola oil	Gluten-free oats	Garlic
Deer	Lentils	Radish	Bell peppers	Raspberries (LG)	Coconut oil	Sorghum	Ginger
Duck	Lima beans	Rutabaga	Bok choy	Strawberries (LG)	Cream (Phase II)	Wild rice	Fennel
Goose	Mung beans	Squash	Broccoli	Apple (MG)	Ghee (clarified butter)	Almond flour	Onion
Lamb	Split peas	Butternut squash	Brussels sprouts	Apricot (MG)	Grapeseed oil	Brown rice flour	Sea salt
Pheasant	Almonds	Spaghetti squash	Cabbage	Cantaloupe (MG)	Macadamia oil	Coconut flour	Black pepper
Pork	Brazil nuts	Acorn squash	Carrots (raw only)	Honeydew (MG)	Olive oil	Garbanzo bean flour	Vanilla
Rabbit	Cashews	Pumpkin	Cauliflower	Kiwi (MG)	Peanut oil		Stevia
Turkey	Chestnuts	Zucchini	Celery	Mango (MG)	Sesame oil		Agave
Veal	Flaxseeds	Yellow summer	Collard greens	Nectarine (MG)			Coconut milk

continues

continued

Animal Proteins (including eggs, meat, and seafood)	Other Proteins (beans, nuts, and legumes)	Starchy Vegetables (acceptable, but eat fewer and combine with fats and proteins)	Nonstarchy Vegetables (eat in unlimited quantities and at every meal and for snacks)	Fruits (LG = Low Glycemic Index; MG = Medium Glycemic Index; HG = High Glycemic Index)	Fats	Grains and Flours (available for Phase II)	Miscellaneous Items
Anchovy	Hazelnuts	Sweet potatoes	Cucumber	Orange (MG)			Almond milk
Bass	Macadamia nuts	Yams	Eggplant	Papaya (MG)			Almond meal
Cod	Pecans		Endive	Peach (MG)			
Grouper	Pumpkin seeds		Green beans	Pear (MG)			
Haddock	Pine nuts		Green onions	Pineapple (MG)			
Halibut	Pistachios		Kale	Plum (MG)			
Herring	Sesame seeds		Lettuce	Banana (HG)			
Mackerel	Sunflower seeds		Mushrooms	Cherries (HG)			
Salmon	Walnuts		Mustard Greens	Dates (HG)			
Sole			Okra	Grapes (HG)			
Tilapia			Onions	Prunes (HG)			
Trout			Peppers	Raisins (HG)			
Walleye			Seaweed	Watermelon (HG)			
Clams			Spinach				
Crab			Swiss chard				
Lobster			Tomatoes				
Mussels			Turnip greens				
Oysters			Watercress				
Scallops							
Shrimp							

One of my favorite ways to prepare a meal is to use tinfoil, parchment paper, and the grill. This method is also very easy to clean up.

1. Choose your protein, vegetable, and spices from the preceding table.

2. Wrap them in some parchment. Put a little olive oil on top.

3. Wrap the parchment-papered fish in some tinfoil to make cooking easier. You want to limit the exposure of your food to the aluminum in the foil, so the parchment paper is a nice barrier.

4. Put them on the grill to cook for 10 to 15 minutes, depending on how well done you like your proteins and veggies.

Meal Ideas

This section shares some meal ideas to help you take the guesswork out of planning what to eat. Many of these meals don't require recipes, and you can have fun finding your favorite way to cook them.

TRUSTY TIP

Focus on foods such as organic fruits and vegetables, grass-fed animals, omega-3 eggs, fresh vegetables, high-fiber fruits, cold-water fish for omega-3 fatty acids, extra-virgin olive oil, fiber, and herbs and spices.

Avoid foods that contain white flour and white sugar; gluten-containing grains; high fructose corn syrup; artificial sweeteners; processed fruit juices; nitrates like what's found in bacon, hot dogs, and processed meats; monosodium glutamate (food additive); fruits or vegetables in non-BPA free cans; hydrogenated oil or trans fats; caffeine; and excess alcohol (no more than three to four glasses per week in Phase II).

Breakfast Ideas

Breakfast truly is the most important meal of the day. You really won't be able to lose weight and keep it off if you skip breakfast. Make sure you include some protein and healthy fats each morning. Here are some suggestions:

• Scrambled eggs with spinach and mushrooms

• Scrambled eggs with tomatoes and asparagus

• Scrambled eggs with smoked salmon and dill

- Scrambled or fried eggs topped with fresh tomato salsa
- Smoked salmon topped with avocado slices and two fried eggs
- Sausage and mushroom frittata
- Grilled tomatoes topped with smoked salmon
- Smoked salmon on cucumber rounds
- Sautéed bell peppers and onion with smoked trout
- Sweet potato hash
- Zucchini pancakes
- Almond pancakes
- Chicken and turkey sausages (organic, nitrate free)
- Roasted apples, cranberries, and walnuts with a sprinkle of cinnamon
- Egg salad
- Muesli—ground flaxseeds and grated walnuts with grated apple or pear and mixed berries

Lunch Ideas

Many of us eat lunch on the run or skip it altogether. Make sure you take the time to consciously eat a healthy lunch. Here are some ideas to get you started:

- Mixed-vegetable salad topped with sunflower seeds or toasted pine nuts and a lean protein (chicken or fish)
- Lettuce wraps filled with chicken salad or shrimp salad
- Lettuce wraps or vegetable salad with chopped cooked chicken or shrimp with chopped red onion, dressed with olive oil, a squeeze of lemon, and salt and pepper
- Bean soup
- Parsnip and cauliflower soup
- Grilled shrimp and scallops topped with tomatillo salsa
- Ratatouille

- Tomatoes stuffed with salmon salad
- Salmon salad over mixed greens
- Fish tacos with cabbage slaw
- Cabbage and sausage meatball soup

Dinner Ideas

Dinner can be difficult when you get home from a busy day and everyone is running in different directions. A little planning ahead will keep you on track preparing quick, healthy dinners and resisting the urge to order out (again). Here are a few suggestions:

- Baked pork loin with braised cabbage and apples
- Grilled shrimp and veggie kebobs
- Sautéed white fish (tilapia, halibut, grouper) with basil and pine nut pesto; serve with roasted asparagus
- Broiled salmon with dill and walnut pesto; serve with broccoli sautéed with garlic and olive oil
- Beef marinara over spaghetti squash; serve with a mixed-green salad
- White bean and kale soup with turkey sausage
- Grilled veal chop served over sautéed lentils and mushrooms; serve with roasted carrots
- Roasted chicken breasts with cauliflower purée and wilted spinach
- Grilled filet mignon with green beans sautéed in olive oil with caramelized onions, slivered almonds, and garlic
- Chicken skewers with peanut sauce; serve with sautéed bok choy and a lentil salad
- Pork loin chops with fennel, tomato, and olive sauce
- Beef and lentil soup
- Chicken and mushroom fajitas in lettuce wraps
- Venison chops with roasted sweet potatoes and sautéed spinach, kale, or Swiss chard
- Prosciutto-wrapped halibut with sage

Snack Ideas

Snacks are an important way to keep your blood sugar stable in between meals. Make sure you always have a few snacks with you at all times so you never get stuck going to the vending machine in desperation. Here are some great snack ideas:

- Apple slices with almond butter
- Pear slices with almond butter
- ½ cup of fresh berries with almonds or walnuts
- Medium-sized whole fruit (apple, pear, orange) and nuts
- Veggies (carrots, celery, cucumber, bell peppers) and hummus
- Veggies and white bean dip
- Canned salmon and white bean salad
- Three-bean salad
- Chopped salad of smoked salmon, hard-boiled egg, and avocado
- Half a sweet potato sprinkled with a little butter and cinnamon and nuts
- Half an avocado and can of sardines
- Guacamole with cucumber and bell pepper slices
- Tomato and cucumber salad with olive oil
- Two-ounce piece of smoked turkey or chicken topped with or without guacamole
- Fresh tomato salsa with sweet potato chips
- Fennel, apple, and walnut salad
- Roasted apples, cranberries, and walnuts with a sprinkle of cinnamon
- Edamame

Phase I: Sample Menus for Four Weeks

Here are sample menus for four weeks of Phase I. They are guidelines only; there are no hard-and-fast rules. Meals that have corresponding recipes in this chapter appear in **bold** type.

Phase I—Week 1

	Monday	Tuesday	Wednesday	Thursday	Friday	Saturday	Sunday
Breakfast	**Spinach and mushroom frittata**	Veggie fritters	Egg salad	**Almond flour pancakes**	Chicken or turkey sausage with eggs	Scrambled eggs with spinach and mushrooms	**Almond flour pancakes**
Snack	Apple slices with almond butter	Orange and walnuts	Pear and handful of almonds	Chopped salad with salmon, hard-boiled egg, and avacado	Half sweet potato with cinnamon, butter, and walnuts	Apple with walnuts	Roasted pears with cinnamon and walnuts
Lunch	Tomatoes stuffed with **salmon salad**	Mixed greens with veggies and chicken or turkey	Lettuce wraps with chicken salad, tomato, and onion	Leftover shrimp and veggies chopped and served in lettuce wraps	Leftover fish tacos with black bean salsa on cabbage leaves	Chicken and sweet potato salad	Scallops with tomato and mushrooms
Snack	Raw veggies with hummus	Guacamole with cucumber	Apple slices with almond butter	Chopped fruit with almonds	Pear slices with almond butter	Turkey and avocado roll	Tomatoes and cucumbers with oil
Dinner	Meatballs in sauce over spaghetti squash	Sautéed white fish with basil and pesto sauce	Grilled shrimp and veggie kabobs	Fish and veggie packets	Roasted chicken breasts with spinach, mushroom, and tomato salad with oil	Stuffed eggplant	Broiled salmon with sautéed broccoli rabe and pine nuts

Phase I—Week 2

	Monday	Tuesday	Wednesday	Thursday	Friday	Saturday	Sunday
Breakfast	Roasted pepper frittata	Smoked salmon on cucumber rounds with dill	Zucchini pancakes	Grilled tomatoes with scrambled eggs	Scrambled eggs with mushrooms and pine nuts	**Almond flour pancakes**	Roasted sweet potato and pear slices with butter and cinnamon
Snack	Chicken salad with apples and pecans	Hard-boiled egg with avocado	Pear slices with almond butter	Veggies and hummus	Berries with almonds or walnuts	Half sweet potato with walnuts	Smoked salmon and hard-boiled egg
Lunch	Turkey rolls with three-bean salad	Cabbage and meatball soup	Mixed greens with veggies and chicken or turkey	**Salmon salad** with white beans over mixed greens	Leftover beef over mixed greens with veggies and oil	Chicken and veggie lettuce wraps	Carrot and ginger soup
Snack	Veggies and hummus	Apple slices with almond butter	Guacamole with cucumber slices	Edamame	Pear with almond butter	Hard-boiled egg and avocado	Berries and nuts
Dinner	Meatballs in sauce over spaghetti squash	**Roasted salmon and zucchini with red pepper sauce**	**Turkey sausage, white bean, and kale soup**	Grilled beef filet with mashed sweet potatoes and sautéed spinach	Baked chicken with steamed green beans	Prosciutto-wrapped halibut with sage and **ratatouille**	**Pork chops with fennel and capers**

Phase I—Week 3

	Monday	Tuesday	Wednesday	Thursday	Friday	Saturday	Sunday
Breakfast	Turkey, dill, and mushroom frittata	Grilled tomatoes topped with smoked salmon	Sautéed spinach and fried eggs	Leftover turkey sausage with chopped apples	Salmon and zucchini fritters	**Almond flour pancakes**	Scrambled eggs with turkey and avocado
Snack	Half baked potato with cinnamon, butter, and nuts	Guacamole with sweet potato chips	Apple with almond butter	Cucumber with smoked salmon	Walnuts and berries	Cucumber with smoked salmon	Chopped pears with raisins and walnuts
Lunch	Shrimp salad in lettuce caps	Tomato and basil soup with spinach salad, chopped egg, and sunflower seeds	Chopped salad with chicken, peas, prosciutto, and tomato over romaine	**Warm tomato and chicken salad**	Leftover steak with sweet potatoes	**Ratatouille**	Minestrone with meat
Snack	Edamame	Celery sticks with almond butter	Veggies and hummus	Apple and almond butter	Three-bean salad	Apple and hard-boiled egg	Celery sticks and almond butter
Dinner	Lamb chops with mint pesto and roasted asparagus	White fish with veggie pockets	Turkey sausage with peppers and onion	Peppered steak with sautéed mushrooms and garlic green beans	Tilapia with chopped tomatoes, capers, and parsley; broccoli on the side	**Sautéed chicken breast with artichokes and peppers**	Lasagna

Phase I–Week 4

	Monday	Tuesday	Wednesday	Thursday	Friday	Saturday	Sunday
Breakfast	Ham and eggs	Tomato and asparagus frittata	Zucchini cakes	Chicken sausage and sweet potato	Veggie fritters	**Almond flour pancakes**	Smoked salmon and chive frittata
Snack	Baked apple with cinnamon	Half baked sweet potato with cinnamon and walnuts	Egg salad	Turkey-wrapped pear slices	Smoked salmon and hard-boiled egg	Leftover ratatouille	Roasted pears and walnuts with cinnamon
Lunch	Mixed greens with veggies and turkey	Leftover veggies and meat	Leek and asparagus soup	Grilled chicken salad over greens with veggies	**Ratatouille**	Leftover steak over greens and veggies	Grilled chicken salad wrapped in lettuce leaves
Snack	Tomato and cucumber salad	Apple and almond butter	Turkey and avocado roll-ups		Veggies and hummus	Salsa and sweet potato chips	Hard-boiled eggs and almonds
Dinner	Slow-cooked garlic veggies and meat	Chicken curry with steamed asparagus	Pork chops with caramelized onions and apples and cauliflower purée	Taco salad over mixed greens	Marinated flank steak with garlic green beans	Baked lemon fish	Pot roast with sweet potatoes and veggies

Recipes

These are recipes for some of the meal suggestions you'll find in the 28-day menu plans. They are very easy to make and taste great. Feel free to improvise and create your own dishes as well.

Super-Fast Weekday Veggie Omelets

I love omelets in the morning, but during the workweek, I don't usually have the time to cook all the ingredients for a great filling. So on the weekend I buy the omelet ingredients for the next week, and I cook five days' worth. Ingredients include the following:

- Spinach, chard, kale, or dandelion greens sliced thinly and sautéed in a tiny bit of olive oil, garlic, and red pepper flakes

- Onions softly simmered in a tiny bit of olive oil and a splash of chicken or veggie broth for about 30 minutes until they are caramelized

- Oven-roasted or grilled vegetables brushed with olive oil, salt, and pepper

- Mushrooms sliced and sautéed in a little bit of olive oil and a handful of chopped parsley thrown in to wilt at the last minute

Make up whatever you like and store it in the refrigerator. Each morning, grab four eggs (I use one whole egg and three whites), whip them up, and pour into a nonstick pan. While the eggs are cooking, measure out ½ cup of the cooked and chopped-up vegetables and put in the microwave for a minute or less to heat through. (Or just toss the veggies in the eggs and scramble it all up.) Fold over your omelet and enjoy.

Spinach and Mushroom Frittata

2 TB. olive oil	Salt and pepper to taste
6 oz. button mushrooms, sliced	½ sack baby spinach
5 eggs	

1. Start out with a 10-inch nonstick skillet over medium heat. Add olive oil, and once hot, add mushrooms. Cook for about 5 minutes, until browned and softened a bit.

2. While mushrooms are cooking, whisk eggs in a small bowl.

3. When mushrooms are done, season with salt and pepper. Add a few handfuls of baby spinach to the skillet and toss until it wilts. (You may need to add a little bit more olive oil to the skillet first.)

4. At this point, preheat your broiler to high.

5. Pour the egg mixture over the mushrooms and spinach. Stir it a few times and cover with a lid. Allow to cook for a few minutes until the bottom is set but still a little runny on top.

6. Place the skillet under the broiler to allow the top to cook. This will take a few minutes. Once it is set on top, remove from your oven. Remember to use a potholder. Then cut into wedges like a pie.

Almond Flour Pancakes

1 cup almond flour	¼ tsp. baking soda
¼ tsp. cinnamon	3 eggs
¼ tsp. pure vanilla	1 TB. water

1. Mix all ingredients into a bowl.

2. Pour batter by ¼ cup onto a hot skillet greased with grapeseed, coconut, or canola oil. When bubbles start to form, cakes are ready to flip.

3. Serve with pure maple syrup or agave nectar. Optional toppings: chopped almonds, flaxseeds, berries, or almond butter.

DID YOU KNOW?

Some "raw/natural" coconut oil cannot be used with high cooking heat. Read the label to confirm if the coconut oil you have is able to be used at high cooking temperatures.

Salmon Salad

2 cans drained or packaged salmon

1 cup cannellini beans (drained and rinsed well if using canned)

1 TB. capers

1 cup artichoke hearts, roughly chopped or quartered

¼ cup kalamata olives, roughly chopped

2 TB. extra-virgin olive oil

2 tsp. red wine vinegar

Fresh ground black pepper and Kosher salt

In a large bowl, mix all ingredients together. Serve.

Roasted Salmon and Zucchini with Red Pepper Sauce

⅓ cup sliced almonds

¼ cup chopped jarred roasted red peppers

1 small clove garlic

1 TB. extra-virgin olive oil

1 TB. sherry vinegar or red-wine vinegar

Kosher salt and pepper

1¼ lb. wild-caught salmon fillet, skinned and cut crosswise into 4 portions

2 medium zucchini, halved lengthwise

2 to 3 TB. olive or grapeseed oil

1 TB. chopped fresh parsley (for garnish)

1. Preheat oven to 375°F. Toast almonds, stirring constantly in a small dry skillet over medium-low heat for 2 to 4 minutes, or until fragrant and lightly browned.

2. Mix almonds, peppers, garlic, extra-virgin olive oil, vinegar, ¼ teaspoon salt, and ¼ teaspoon pepper in a food processor until smooth; set aside.

3. Drizzle salmon and zucchini on both sides with olive oil, then sprinkle with salt and pepper. Place in the oven and roast, turning once halfway through, until salmon is just cooked through and zucchini is soft and browned, about 5 minutes per side. When cool enough to handle, slice the zucchini into ½-inch pieces.

4. Toss in a bowl with half of reserved sauce. Divide zucchini among four plates along with a piece of salmon topped with some of remaining sauce. Garnish with parsley.

Turkey Sausage, White Bean, and Kale Soup

1 onion, diced

1 TB. olive oil

1 clove garlic, minced

4 cooked turkey wine sausages

Salt and pepper

1 L organic chicken stock

1 bunch kale, well-washed, de-stalked, and roughly chopped

1 (28-oz.) can Great Northern beans, drained and rinsed

1. Sauté onion in olive oil until translucent. Add garlic and cook for 1 minute, then add turkey wine sausages and let cook for another few minutes. Sprinkle in some salt and pepper. Add chicken stock and bring to a gentle simmer.

2. Stir in kale and cook for about 15 minutes before adding Great Northern beans. Simmer until kale is tender. Taste and correct for seasoning.

Pork Chops with Fennel and Capers

¼ cup olive oil

4 boneless (2-inch-thick) pork chops (about 2 lb. total)

Salt and pepper

2 fennel bulbs with fronds, thinly sliced (about 8 oz. or 2 cups)

2 large shallots, thinly sliced

⅔ cup chopped fresh flat-leaf parsley, divided in half

½ cup dry white wine or vermouth

6 plum tomatoes, chopped

½ cup low-sodium vegetable broth

2 TB. butter

2 TB. capers

1. In a large, heavy skillet, heat olive oil over high heat. Season pork chops with salt and pepper. Add pork to the pan and brown on both sides, about 4 minutes each. Remove pork from the pan, cover loosely with foil, and set aside.

2. Add fennel, shallots, and ⅓ cup parsley to the pan and cook over medium heat until they begin to brown, about 5 minutes. Add white wine. Using a wooden spoon, scrape the brown bits off the bottom of the pan. Add tomatoes and vegetable broth to the pan, and stir. Add pork back into the pan, nestling chops between fennel and tomatoes so they are mostly submerged in pan juices. Cook until fennel is tender and the pork is done, about 12 to 15 minutes.

3. Place pork on a serving dish. To finish sauce, add butter, remaining parsley, capers, and salt and pepper to taste. Stir to combine. Pour over pork chops and serve.

Warm Chicken and Tomato Salad

¼ cup olive oil and to taste

1 red onion

1 clove crushed garlic

2 chopped organic chicken breasts, boneless and skinless

Salt and pepper

2 cups cherry tomatoes

Mixed organic greens or baby spinach to taste

Balsamic vinegar to taste

1. Place olive oil, onion, and garlic into frying pan and heat for 3 to 4 minutes, until onion is just soft.

2. Add chicken, salt, and pepper to pan and continue to stir until chicken is almost cooked through. Add cherry tomatoes to chicken and onion mixture and cook until tomatoes are warm and soft. Remove from heat and pour mixture over mixed greens. Dress with olive oil and balsamic vinegar before serving.

Ratatouille

1 to 2 TB. oil

2 chopped onions

3 cloves crushed garlic

1 medium eggplant, peeled and chopped

2 large zucchini, peeled and chopped

2 TB. tomato paste

2 cups chopped tomatoes

1 tsp. coriander

1 tsp. dried basil

Salt and pepper to taste

1. In a large pan, heat oil, onions, and garlic until onion is soft.

2. Add eggplant and zucchini, then cover and simmer on low for 20 minutes. Add tomato paste, tomatoes, coriander, basil, salt, and pepper to the pan and continue to cook for another 20 to 30 minutes until vegetables are tender. Serve.

Sautéed Chicken Breast with Artichokes and Peppers

4 tsp. extra-virgin olive oil

4 boneless, skinless chicken breasts (about 6 oz. each)

Kosher salt and freshly ground black pepper

1 onion, halved and sliced

4 cloves garlic, smashed

2 sprigs fresh thyme, leaves stripped

1½ cups jarred marinated artichokes, drained and patted dry

½ cup jarred roasted red peppers, sliced into strips

1 cup chicken broth, homemade or low-sodium canned

1 to 2 TB. unsalted butter

¼ cup flat-leaf parsley leaves

1. Preheat oven to 400°F.

2. Heat a large skillet over medium-high heat; add extra-virgin olive oil. Season chicken with salt and pepper to taste. Lay chicken skinned-side down in the skillet and cook, turning once, until golden, about 4 minutes per side. Transfer chicken to a baking dish or roasting pan and bake until firm to the touch, about 10 minutes.

3. Meanwhile, add onion, garlic, and thyme to the skillet and season with salt and pepper. Cook, stirring occasionally, until brown, about 5 minutes. Add the artichokes and peppers and cook until brown, about 3 minutes. Stir with a wooden spoon to scrape up browned bits from the bottom of the pan.

4. Add chicken broth and bring mixture to a full boil. Simmer until the sauce thickens and season with salt and pepper. Whisk in butter and add parsley. Pour sauce over chicken and serve.

The Least You Need to Know

- The first 30 days of Phase I will remove many of the foods people are most sensitive to: grains and dairy.
- You won't lose weight if you skip breakfast.
- Make sure you always have portable snack options with you so you can maintain a steady blood sugar.
- Use parchment paper when you cook with tinfoil to limit the exposure of your food to the foil.

Phase II: Eating for Optimal Health

In This Chapter

- What to watch for as you start Phase II
- Questions answered about alcohol
- Sample menus
- Recipes

Welcome to Phase II! Hopefully, you were able to enjoy a number of the recipes in Phase I. Phase II gives you more latitude with the addition of full-fat dairy and some gluten-free whole grains. There's a variety in the recipes. My hope is that you enjoy this way of eating and can maintain it as your lifestyle.

What to Watch for as You Start Phase II

Remember the 80/20 rule: after you heal your metabolism, if you maintain your healthy eating habits 80 percent of the time, you should be able to relax and eat something less than optimal occasionally (or 20 percent of the time). You might notice that certain foods you used to enjoy really don't appeal to you now. The reality is that they probably never did really agree with you; you were just generally feeling badly and didn't notice it.

Watch closely how you feel with the addition of dairy and grains. If you find that you're gaining weight and getting headaches, sinus congestion, bloating, diarrhea, rashes, or constipation, stop eating both the grains and dairy. You can then try adding them back, one at a time—grains first and then dairy—and see whether you can pinpoint your specific sensitivity.

You may also enjoy a little alcohol during this phase. As with the addition of the other new foods, if you start gaining weight, stop drinking alcohol for a little while longer until your metabolism heals a little more.

What About Alcohol?

As you move to Phase II, you can add a small amount of alcohol back into your diet. Optimally, to maintain the best health and hormone balance, you should not consume alcohol at all. It's high in sugar, disturbs your sleep patterns, and stresses your liver. That being said, it's often part of your social life and can be consumed in moderation.

If you're truly having difficulty losing weight, alcohol might be something you need to give up until you reach your goal weight or size. Your liver and metabolism might be too stressed to handle it.

If you choose to drink alcohol, keep in mind some basic rules that will limit its negative effects on you. First, alcohol shuts down your body's ability to make natural human growth hormone (HGH). Because you make the majority of your HGH in the first 90 minutes of sleep, it makes sense not to have alcohol in your system when you go to bed for the night. If you're going to drink alcohol, do so around happy hour time so your body has a chance to clear the alcohol before you go to bed.

Also, keep in mind that many of the drinks that contain alcohol also contain a ton of sugar. Switch to drinks that don't use a lot of sugar. For instance, there are several flavored vodkas on the market. You can use flavored vodka, such as raspberry, with club soda and lime. You will significantly limit the sugar, and the acidity in the lime will reduce the insulin response. If you drink beer, look for a gluten-free variety because most beers are full of gluten. If you drink wine, red wine has more antioxidants. However, you can do a small amount of white wine with club soda as a spritzer to limit the amount of alcohol you're taking in as well.

Sample Menus

I have included some sample menus for Phase II. Remember that you can use any of the Phase I meals at any point in Phase II. Again, the choices in **bold** have recipes listed at the end of the chapter.

Phase II—Week 1

	Monday	Tuesday	Wednesday	Thursday	Friday	Saturday	Sunday
Breakfast	Chicken sausage with scrambled eggs	Ezekial wrap with almond butter and fruit	Gluten-free oatmeal	Smoked salmon and scrambled eggs in Ezekial wrap	**Fruit and nut granola**	Almond flour pancakes	Omelet with roasted veggies
Snack	**High-protein smoothie**	Cucumbers with hummus and olives	Pear with almond butter	Fennel and apple and walnut salad	Hard-boiled egg and avocado	Mixed berries with Greek yogurt	**High-protein smoothie**
Lunch	Roasted asparagus and quinoa salad	Grilled chicken salad over mixed greens	Chopped veggie salad with chicken	Turkey Cobb salad	Leftover chicken and three-bean salad	Salmon with **lentil salad**	Salmon with tomatoes and avocado in Ezekial wrap
Snack	Sweet potato chips with salsa	Apple and walnuts	Veggies and Greek yogurt dip	Edamame	Veggies and hummus	Half sweet potato with nuts and cinnamon	Apple and cashews
Dinner	Chicken and broccoli stir-fry with brown rice	**Pork chops with caramelized apples and onions**	Ground turkey and sauce over spaghetti squash	Lemon chicken sautéed with spinach and brown rice	Roasted salmon and zucchini with red pepper sauce	Stuffed peppers with brown rice and turkey	Roast beef with horse-radish, mashed sweet potatoes, and asparagus

Phase II—Week 2

	Monday	Tuesday	Wednesday	Thursday	Friday	Saturday	Sunday
Breakfast	Gluten-free granola with Greek yogurt and berries	Egg salad	Gluten-free oatmeal	Almond flour pancakes	Ezekial wrap with almond butter and fruit	Turkey and avocado omelet	Chicken sausage, roasted apples, cranberries, walnuts, and cinnamon
Snack	Chopped smoked salmon and egg and avocado salad	Mixed nuts and dried cranberries	Pear with almond butter	**High-protein smoothie**	Greek yogurt and berries	Apple, walnut, and fennel salad	Cucumber and guacamole
Lunch	Chicken salad–stuffed tomato	Turkey and spinach in Ezekial wrap with mustard	Leftover chicken and mixed greens with veggies	Leftover shrimp in lettuce leaves	Spinach salad with chicken, egg, tomato, and sunflower seeds	Tilapia with pesto, brown rice, and asparagus	Seared scallops and quinoa salad
Snack	Turkey and veggie roll-ups	Veggies and white bean dip	Veggies and Greek yogurt dip	Turkey and veggie roll-ups	Half sweet potato with cinnamon and nuts	Kale chips and dip	Edamame
Dinner	Fish tacos in cabbage leaf with roasted sweet potatoes	**Jerk chicken with mango salsa** and quinoa salad	Shrimp with brown rice, tomato, and basil	**Mediterra-nean chicken with Tzatziki sauce**	Pork chops with green beans	Sautéed chicken breast with artichokes and peppers	Chicken and brown rice soup

Phase II—Week 3

	Monday	Tuesday	Wednesday	Thursday	Friday	Saturday	Sunday
Breakfast	Chicken sausage with scrambled eggs	Ezekial wrap with almond butter and sliced fruit	Sliced tomato, salmon, and avocado	Granola with berries and Greek yogurt	Gluten-free oatmeal	Almond flour pancakes	Frittata with asparagus and tomato
Snack	**High-protein smoothie**	Carrot, raisin, and walnut salad	Apple and almond butter	Apple and small piece of chicken	Berries and Greek yogurt	Egg salad	Kale chips and dip
Lunch	Mixed greens, chicken, and veggies	Chicken over Greek salad	Quinoa salad and leftover shrimp	Hummus and veggies in Ezekial wrap	Leftover chicken and ratatouille	Leftover salmon on spinach salad	Turkey and avocado Ezekial wraps
Snack	Turkey and veggie roll-ups	Veggies and hummus	Veggies and Greek yogurt dip	Pear and almond butter	Half sweet potato with walnuts and cinnamon	Edamame	**High-protein smoothie**
Dinner	**Mediterranean chicken with Tzatziki sauce**	Grilled shrimp and veggie kabobs with brown rice	Fajitas	Chicken and ratatouille	Broiled salmon with lemon and dill; broccoli in garlic and oil	**Tuna and spinach salad**	Grilled marinated flank steak with green beans

Phase II—Week 4

	Monday	Tuesday	Wednesday	Thursday	Friday	Saturday	Sunday
Breakfast	Gluten-free oatmeal	**High-protein smoothie**	Smoked salmon and chive omelet	Granola and berries with Greek yogurt	Veggie fritters	Chicken sausage with scrambled eggs	Asparagus and goat cheese omelet
Snack	**High-protein smoothie**	Apple and almond butter	Orange and walnuts	Pear and turkey slices	Veggies and hummus	Apple and almond butter	Roasted apples with cinnamon
Lunch	Leftover steak and mixed greens with veggies	Egg salad with lettuce in Ezekial wrap	Shrimp salad with leftovers on lettuce wrap	Leftover soup	Salmon salad on tomato	Black bean soup	Chicken salad with brown rice
Snack	Veggies with hummus	Leftover turkey and veggies	Veggies and Greek yogurt dip	Carrot, raisin, and walnut salad	Half sweet potato with walnuts and cinnamon	Turkey and veggie roll-ups	Cucumber with guacamole slices
Dinner	Roasted turkey breast with baked sweet potatoes and broccoli	Shrimp, snow pea, and red pepper stir-fry with brown rice	White bean and kale soup with turkey sausage	Roasted chicken with asparagus	Trout and veggie pockets	**Thai chicken salad**	Filet mignon with **lentil salad**

Recipes

The following recipes will jump-start your Phase II plan.

Gets-the-Job-Done Daily Oatmeal

¼ cup organic rolled oats (not instant)

1 cup water

Pinch sea salt

1 heaping TB. or scoop plain brown rice protein powder (unsweetened, organic)

1 to 2 TB. ground flaxseed meal (preferably organic)

¼ cup frozen or fresh wild or organic blueberries

1 TB. slivered almonds

Cinnamon to taste

1 to 2 packets stevia (optional)

Splash almond milk (I use unsweetened)

1. Put oats, water, and sea salt in a bowl and microwave on high for 2 minutes.

2. Add protein powder, flaxseed meal, blueberries, almonds, cinnamon, and stevia and stir.

3. Splash almond milk to your desired consistency and stir. Enjoy!

Wheat- and Gluten-Free Breakfast Peanut Butter Quesadillas

1 TB. nut butter of your choice (smooth butters spread easier— try almond butter)

1 Ezekial wrap (available at Whole Foods and other health food stores in the refrigerator or freezer)

1 tsp. flaxseeds

½ banana, apple, or pear, sliced

Drizzle agave nectar

1. Spread nut butter on one half of Ezekial wrap.

2. Sprinkle with flaxseeds, then lay fruit slices on top. Drizzle with a little bit of agave nectar.

3. Fold over and cut in half. Serve.

Fruit and Nut Granola

Cooking spray

3 cups old-fashioned oats

½ cup chopped walnuts

½ cup chopped almonds

½ cup chopped pecans

¼ cup flaxseed

½ cup honey

¼ tsp salt

¼ tsp cinnamon

½ cup dried fruit (raisins, cranberries, cherries, or chopped apricots)

1. Preheat oven to 300°F. Coat a large baking sheet with cooking spray. In a bowl, combine all ingredients, mixing well to coat everything with honey. Spread on the baking sheet and bake until golden brown, stirring occasionally, about 30 minutes.

2. Cool completely on a wire rack. This can be stored in the refrigerator in an airtight container for about 2 weeks. Serve with milk or on plain yogurt with fresh berries.

TRUSTY TIP

All of the nuts in this recipe provide protein and a variety of healthy fats and minerals, such as magnesium and potassium. They also keep blood sugar stable, reduce the risk for heart disease, and can help control appetite and weight. The cinnamon also helps regulate blood sugar.

High-Protein Smoothie

1 cup unsweetened almond milk

½ cup frozen organic berries or cherries

1 to 2 packets stevia

1 scoop rice protein powder

1 TB. flaxseeds or flaxseed meal

Ice cubes, if desired

Toss all ingredients in a blender and blend till smooth. Serve.

Lentil Salad

10 to 20 cherry tomatoes

Olive oil

2 cups lentils

Juice of 1 lemon

1 bay leaf

3 cloves crushed garlic

1 bunch parsley, chopped

1 large red onion, chopped

1 cup pitted olives

4 oz. Parmesan cheese, grated

1. Preheat oven to 250°F. Place cherry tomatoes on baking tray with small amount of olive oil and bake for 40 minutes.

2. Place lentils in a pan with lemon juice, bay leaf, garlic, and enough water to cover them. Cover and cook for 40 minutes.

3. Drain lentils and transfer to serving bowl. Mix in cherry tomatoes, parsley, red onion, olives, and small amount of olive oil. Top with Parmesan cheese and serve.

Pan-Seared Pork Chops with Caramelized Apples and Onions

2 tsp. olive oil

4 pork loin chops (about 4 oz. each)

Salt and freshly ground black pepper to taste

1 medium yellow onion, peeled, halved, and thinly sliced

1 sprig fresh thyme, or ½ tsp. dried

3 tart apples, peeled (optional), cored, and sliced

1 cup apple cider

1. Heat olive oil in a large skillet over medium-high heat. Season pork chops with salt and pepper and sear them on both sides until just cooked through, about 4 to 6 minutes per side. (Thinner chops will take less time, while thicker chops will take a bit longer.) Transfer pork chops to a platter and keep warm.

2. In the same pan, add onion and thyme and turn the heat to medium. Season with salt and pepper and cook until onions begin to wilt, about 3 minutes.

3. Turn the heat to high, and cook until onions are golden brown. Add apples and apple cider and cook until cider has reduced and slightly thickened and apples are tender, about 6 minutes. Remove thyme sprig. Top pork chops with apple-onion mixture and serve.

Jerk Chicken Breasts with Mango Salsa

2 tsp. extra-virgin olive oil, plus some for drizzling

1½ tsp. ground allspice

½ tsp. dried basil

½ tsp. ground cinnamon

½ tsp. ground nutmeg

1½ tsp. dried thyme

½ tsp. cayenne pepper

1½ tsp. light brown sugar

Salt and freshly ground black pepper

2 chicken breasts

1 ripe mango, peeled and diced

1 small red bell pepper, seeded and diced

1 jalapeño pepper, seeded and finely chopped

¼ seedless cucumber, peeled and chopped

1 lime, juiced

1. Heat extra-virgin olive oil in a large skillet over medium heat. In a mixing bowl, combine allspice, basil, cinnamon, nutmeg, thyme, cayenne pepper, brown sugar, salt, and pepper and mix to combine them. Cover chicken breasts in spice mixture and drizzle with extra-virgin olive oil. Add chicken breasts to the skillet and cook about 5 minutes on both sides or until cooked all the way through; there shouldn't be any pink in the middle.

2. While chicken cooks, in a small bowl, combine mango, bell pepper, jalapeño pepper, cucumber, and lime juice.

3. When chicken breasts are done, transfer them to a serving platter, then cover with mango salsa. Serve.

Mediterranean Chicken with Tzatziki Sauce

½ tsp. dried oregano

¼ cup olive oil

2 TB. balsamic vinegar

2 garlic cloves, divided

1 lb. chicken breast, preferably organic, cut into strips

1 cup plain Greek yogurt

½ cup grated cucumber, squeeze out excess water

Juice of ½ lemon

Freshly ground black pepper and Kosher salt to season

1. Mix oregano, olive oil, balsamic vinegar, and 1 garlic clove (minced or passed through a garlic press) together. Pour over chicken and marinate for at least 1 hour. Then cook by either grilling or broiling in the oven.

2. In a bowl, add remaining garlic clove (I like to grate it), Greek yogurt, cucumber, lemon juice, pepper, and salt. Mix well.

3. Serve chicken with sauce or stuff into a whole-grain pita.

Tuna and Spinach Salad

Baby spinach leaves

½ cup drained olives

1 cucumber, chopped

1 medium onion, chopped

8 to 10 cherry tomatoes, cut in half

1 (6-oz.) can solid light tuna in water, drained

2 hard-boiled eggs

Salt and pepper to taste

Olive oil to taste

Balsamic vinegar to taste

1. Toss together baby spinach, olives, cucumber, onion, and cherry tomatoes. Place tuna on top of greens.

2. Garnish with hard-boiled eggs, salt, pepper, olive oil, and vinegar. Serve.

Thai Chicken Salad

2 boneless, skinless chicken breasts

2 TB. teriyaki sauce

Mixed greens to fill plate

½ avocado

½ cup chopped cilantro

¼ cup chopped peanuts

6 chopped scallions

1 tsp. red pepper flakes

1 cup chopped cucumber

Salt and pepper to taste

Olive oil to taste

1. Marinate chicken in teriyaki sauce in the refrigerator for 30 to 60 minutes. Remove from marinade and grill.

2. Place mixed greens on plates and add sliced avocado, cilantro, peanuts, scallions, red pepper flakes, cucumber, salt, and pepper. Place chicken on top of salads, drizzle with olive oil, and serve.

The Least You Need to Know

- If you are sensitive to grains, adding them back in Phase II might cause weight gain. Watch how you feel for the first few times you eat grains.

- Remember the 80/20 rule. You should have some leeway to be flexible with your eating habits 20 percent of the time if you're careful the other 80 percent.

- If you choose to drink alcohol, make sure your drinks don't have a lot of added sugars. Use club soda and fruit slices as your mixers.

My Personal Action Plan

In This Chapter

- Understanding the difference between fat and muscle
- The information you need to build your personal action plan
- Sample action plans for specific groups

The seven principles of the hormone weight-loss diet are key to balancing hormones and maintaining a healthy weight. But how do you apply these principles to your daily life? How do you adapt them for your particular needs and goals? For example, let's say you're 30 years old, female, and want to wear clothes four sizes smaller than your present size 16. Your approach would obviously be different than your neighbor's who is 50 years old and only wants to drop down one size. This chapter gives you the information you need to build a diet plan for your particular circumstances.

Muscle vs. Fat

You might have noticed that I don't discuss calories or calorie counting regarding this diet. I believe that if you're eating whole foods without artificial sweeteners, high fructose corn syrup, refined carbohydrates, and trans fats, you'll heal your metabolism and your appetite. Then your body will be able to naturally regulate the amount of food you consume. I also don't talk about weight or losing a certain number of pounds. This is because weight can be deceiving. Here's why.

The approach used most often to determine whether calorie counting is working (other than the bathroom scale) is the widely used *body mass index* (*BMI*), a measure of how tall you are in relation to your weight. It's helpful as a general guidance tool. However, its major shortcoming is that it doesn't take into account what your weight is composed of: muscle or fat.

> **DEFINITION**
>
> **Body mass index (BMI)** is an approximation for human body fat based on an individual's weight and height. BMI does not actually measure the percentage of body fat; it's the individual's body weight divided by the square of his or her height.

For example, the following two people have the same BMI: a male who is 5 foot 6 inches and weighs 160 pounds with 15 percent body fat versus a woman who is 5 foot 6 inches and weighs 150 pounds with 40 percent body fat. The male has a significantly higher amount of lean muscle mass and therefore a much higher metabolism, which makes a huge difference in maintaining a healthy weight.

Many of my patients complain that when they diet they do "all the right things," yet the scale doesn't move. This can actually be a good thing, especially if you're doing interval and resistance training, because you're building muscle mass. And muscle weighs more but takes up less space than fat.

If you're only watching the scale, you might not see much of a change. The number on the scale might even go up. This can be incredibly discouraging if you don't understand what's going on. Because muscle takes up less space than fat, you should start to see a difference in the way your clothes fit. Focus more on size than on weight. The more muscle you have, the higher your metabolism and the more calories you burn every minute of the day, regardless of what you're doing.

Action Plan Worksheets

To get started in your hormone weight-loss program, go to Appendix D and locate the action plan worksheet. You can also download it at my website, www. DrAliciaStanton.com.

I highly recommend that you take the time to take the measurements suggested on the action plan worksheet and to have someone take a photograph of you from the front and the side. This is important because you might not notice subtle changes that will appear in photographs taken later. After 30, 60, and 90 days, the measurements and pictures will be helpful in documenting your progress.

Also, make sure you take the quiz in Chapter 15 to find out whether your hormones are balanced. Information is provided at the end of this chapter regarding low thyroid, metabolic syndrome, men's health, and women's health. If you have concerns in those areas after taking the quiz, consider supplementation based on suggestions in those sections. Next, find the following section that applies to you and the corresponding worksheet.

Children

Adequate nutrition plays an important role during childhood, providing the groundwork for growth, development, and health. Unfortunately, the current epidemic of childhood obesity is setting up many children for a lifetime of high risk for hormone imbalance, chronic disease, and eating disorders.

During the school-age years, the growth of children is steady but not as rapid as it was in infancy or as it will be in adolescence. Children usually have occasional spurts of growth that coincide with periods of increased appetite and food intake. During periods of slower growth, children's appetite and intake should decrease. Keep in mind, a child's pattern of growth over time is much more important than any single measurement.

Monitoring childhood obesity can be difficult because there's a natural increase in BMI at some points during childhood, usually just prior to growth spurts. This shouldn't be mistaken for obesity.

If you're a parent, make sure that your child has access to healthy food choices, including fruits, vegetables, proteins, and healthy fats. Limit exposure to artificial sweeteners, refined carbohydrates, trans fats, and high fructose corn syrup. And create plenty of opportunities for your child to get regular exercise.

Your child's clothing size now: _____

Your child's ideal clothing size: _____

Losing Sizes

If you want your child to lose one or two sizes, implement Phase I for 30 days (see Chapter 20). After 30 days, move your child to Phase II and slowly add some gluten-free grains back into the diet (see Chapter 21). If you find that he or she is gaining weight or getting larger again, go back to Phase I for another 30 days.

If your child needs to lose three or more sizes, he or she should remain on Phase I for 60 to 90 days.

Success and Maintenance

Make sure that your child continues to follow the seven principles of the diet. If you find that he or she is gaining weight or increasing in size again, repeat Phase I for 30 days.

Teenagers

Adolescence is a time of profound biological, social, and emotional change that bridges the gap from childhood into adulthood. The adolescent experiences many of the same things that he or she did as a toddler: development of personal identity; separation from parents; and adjustment to a new body that is changing in shape, size, and physical capacity. These changes have direct effects on nutritional needs. Their dramatic physical growth and development significantly increase their needs for energy, protein, vitamins, and minerals.

However, a teenager's struggle for independence might lead to the development of compromising eating behaviors, such as starvation dieting, meal skipping, eating a lot of junk foods, and using unconventional nutritional supplementation such as extreme herbal weight-loss products or bodybuilding products found over the counter. These behaviors can damage the metabolism and lead to lifelong issues with weight, inflammation, hormone imbalance, and chronic disease.

As much as 50 percent of a teenager's ideal body weight is gained and almost half of adult peak bone mass is accrued during adolescence. By age 18, more than 90 percent of adult skeletal mass has been formed.

In females, most of the weight gain comes three to six months after an increase in height. From the age of around 10 to when they start menstruating, they might gain an average of 18 pounds per year and gain an average of 14 more pounds during the latter half of adolescence. Females experience on average a 44 percent increase in lean body mass (muscle) and a 120 percent increase in body fat during puberty. This causes the average lean body mass in females to fall from 80 percent to 74 percent and the average body fat to increase from 16 percent to 27 percent when they're fully mature. This is important because research has shown a level of 17 percent body fat is required for menstruation to occur and 25 percent body fat is required for the development and maintenance of regular ovulatory cycles.

For males, peak weight gain coincides with the timing of peak height increase and peak muscle mass accumulation. During peak weight gain, adolescent males put on an average gain of 20 pounds per year. Body fat decreases in adolescent males to about 12 percent at the end of puberty.

As with children, it's sometimes difficult to determine whether a teenager is overweight and on the road to obesity or getting ready for a growth spurt. The smartest move is to continue encouraging whole foods, regularly timed meals and snacks, adequate sleep, and adequate activity, and to limit refined carbohydrates, trans fats, artificial sweeteners, and high fructose corn syrup. If, however, there is a significant amount of excess weight, focus on encouraging healthy habits rather than discussing dieting.

The following action plan is designed for the teen to fill out and use:

My size now: _____

The size I want to be: _____

Losing Sizes

If you're trying to lose one or two sizes, do Phase I for 30 days. After 30 days, you can move to Phase II and slowly add some gluten-free grains back into your diet. If you find that you're gaining weight or getting larger again, go back to Phase I for another 30 days.

If you want to lose three or more sizes, remain on Phase I for 60 to 90 days, depending on how many sizes you would like to lose. When you're at your desired size, slowly start adding a few of the gluten-free grains into your diet and see how you do. You might find that your progress slows with the addition of the grains. If that happens, remove them from your diet again. You should also limit your servings of fruit to one serving per day until your metabolism is more stable. Focus your meals and snacks on vegetables, proteins, and healthy fats.

Success and Maintenance

Continue following the seven principles of the diet. If you find that you're gaining weight or increasing in size again, repeat Phase I for 30 days.

The 20s

This is a time when many young men and women "push it to the limit." Whether it's school stress and all-nighters, a job with irregular hours, or new friends and late parties, there's always something going on. It's easy to eat convenience foods on the run or skip meals. The danger is that because you're young, your metabolism might not be significantly damaged yet, and you might not notice weight gain or other symptoms of poor nutrition like fatigue or acne.

The U.S. Department of Agriculture has done research showing that less than half of young men and women get even 50 percent of the U.S. recommended daily allowance (RDA) of many vitamins and minerals. This is particularly scary because the U.S. RDA levels are only adequate to prevent significant nutritional diseases such as rickets and scurvy. They don't provide adequate protection for optimal health.

Adequate nutrients are critical at this stage in life because poor nutrition (either overeating or undereating) can create later problems with metabolism and conception.

The good news is that if your metabolism is damaged now and you're overweight, you're young enough that by carefully adhering to the principles of the hormone weight-loss diet, you should be able to heal your metabolism more easily than if you wait until you're older.

Make sure that you're getting enough sleep. It might be easy to "push through" the fatigue when you're young, but the bad effects of inadequate sleep add up. Make sure you're eating every two to three hours and focusing on lean proteins, vegetables, and high-fiber fruits and healthy fats. Eliminate refined carbohydrates, trans fats, high fructose corn syrup, caffeine, and artificial sweeteners.

My size now: _____

The size I want to be: _____

Losing Sizes

If you want to lose one to two sizes, you should do Phase I for the first 30 days and consider switching to Phase II. If, as you switch to Phase II, you notice that you're gaining weight or increasing in size again, go back to Phase I. Also, you should do interval training to increase your lean muscle mass and metabolism.

If you want to lose three or more sizes, remain on Phase I for 60 to 90 days depending on how many sizes you would like to lose. When you're at your desired size, slowly start adding a few gluten-free grains into your diet and see how you do. You might find that your progress slows with the addition of the grains. If that happens, remove them from your diet again. You should also limit your servings of fruit to one serving per day until your metabolism is more stable. Focus your meals and snacks on vegetables, proteins, and healthy fats.

Success and Maintenance

Continue following the seven principles of the diet. If you find that you're gaining weight or increasing in size again, repeat Phase I for 30 days. Also, keep a very close eye on how much sleep you're getting and what your stress levels are.

Women (Age 30–55)

This is the time when many women are focusing on raising children, building careers, and potentially caring for elderly parents. These years can be among the most amazing and fulfilling times in your life. However, they can be significantly stressful years as well. Depending on how you eat, exercise, sleep, and generally take care of yourself, you might have a metabolism that is healthy or one that needs work.

Hormonal shifts related to reproduction, diet, and stress have the biggest impact on the needs of your body. After menopause, loss of estrogen leads to an increase in abdominal fat, among other things. Menopause is associated with, but not necessarily the cause of, weight gain and decreased muscle mass. By focusing on the principles of the diet, it's possible to maintain adequate muscle mass and good hormone balance.

My size now: _____

The size I want to be: _____

Losing Sizes

If you want to lose one to two sizes, you should do Phase I for the first 30 days and then consider switching to Phase II. If, as you switch to Phase II, you notice that you're gaining weight or increasing in size again, go back to Phase I. Also, you should be doing interval training to increase your lean muscle mass and metabolism.

If you want to lose three or more sizes, remain on Phase I for 60 to 90 days, depending on how many sizes you'd like to lose. When you're at your desired size, slowly start adding a few gluten-free grains into your diet and see how you do. You might find that your progress slows with the addition of the grains. If that happens, remove them from your diet again. You should also limit your servings of fruit to one serving per day until your metabolism is more stable. Focus your meals and snacks on vegetables, proteins, and healthy fats.

You might want to consider supplementation to help increase your insulin sensitivity and stabilize your adrenals. You should focus on interval training and strength training, making sure to scale the exercises appropriately to your ability.

Success and Maintenance

After you reach your desired size, continue to follow all the principles of the diet. It's going to be important for you to limit stress and cortisol demand. Also, it's important for you to get adequate sleep and limit your exposure to toxins. If you find that you're continually having trouble with maintaining your desired weight or size, consider hormone testing to see whether there's an imbalance in your hormones.

If you have any health issues such as metabolic syndrome, low thyroid, PMS, or polycystic ovarian syndrome, or you are on any hormone therapy, please see the end of this chapter for supplementation information. Remember, information on adrenal supplementation and sleep is in Chapter 16, and information on detoxification is in Chapter 12.

Men (Age 35–55)

This is an important time for men. Your testosterone peaks in your 20s and, from now on, you'll have a small but yearly decline in your natural testosterone production. Doing things such as eating appropriately, managing your stress, and exercising now will make a huge difference as you enter your 50s and beyond.

For many men, this is the time when they're building a career and raising a family. They're young enough that it's easy to put their own health aside and "burn the candle at both ends" trying to get ahead. It might seem like it makes sense in the short term. However, in the long term, it is a recipe for disaster.

If you're overweight now, you're more likely to produce extra estrogen, which will work against the testosterone you have. This places you at an increased risk for depression, prostate problems, heart disease, diabetes, and decreased fertility. It's important to focus on the seven principles of this diet plan, increase your lean muscle mass, and heal your metabolism so you can reduce the risk of these complications in the future. By doing strength interval training, you'll enhance your natural production of testosterone and human growth hormone (HGH). As you lose belly fat, you will reduce the conversion of your testosterone to estrogen, which will move you toward improved hormone balance.

My size now: _____

The size I want to be: _____

Losing Sizes

If you want to lose one to two sizes, you should do Phase I of the diet for the first 30 days and consider switching to Phase II. If, as you switch to Phase II, you notice that you're gaining weight or increasing in size again, go back to Phase I. Also, you should be doing interval training to increase your lean muscle mass and metabolism.

If you want to lose three or more sizes, remain on Phase I for 60 to 90 days, depending on how many sizes you'd like to lose. When you're at your desired size, slowly start adding a few of the gluten-free grains into your diet and see how you do. You might find that your progress slows with the addition of the grains. If that happens, remove them from your diet again. You should also limit your servings of fruit to one serving per day until your metabolism is more stable. Focus your meals and snacks on vegetables, proteins, and healthy fats.

You might want to consider supplementation to help increase your insulin sensitivity and stabilize your adrenals. You should focus on interval training and strength training, making sure to scale the exercises appropriately to your ability.

Success and Maintenance

After you reach your desired size, continue to follow all the principles of the diet. It's going to be important for you to limit stress and cortisol demand. Also, it's important for you to get adequate sleep and limit your exposure to toxins. If you find that you're continually having trouble with maintaining your desired weight or size, consider hormone testing to see whether there is an imbalance and your hormones.

55-Plus

If you're age 55 or older, the reality is that you're in the second half of your life, and you want to make sure that you're in a good place. The bad news is that if you've been able to "get by" with minimal effort on your diet, and it has not always been the best kind of diet, you might be in for a rude awakening. Now, in order to maintain a healthy amount of lean muscle mass and body fat, you need to pay attention to what you eat and how you live.

Adequate sleep and stress management are paramount at this point, because you don't have the reserve that you used to. Because of hormone shifts, it's much easier to gain fat, especially abdominal fat, at this point. Abdominal fat tends to increase the amount of available estrogen in both men and women, and it increases inflammation. Adhering to all the principles of this diet is important, especially now.

My size now: _____

The size I want to be: _____

Losing Sizes

If you want to lose one to two sizes, you should do Phase I for the first 30 days and then consider switching to Phase II. If, as you switch to Phase II, you notice that you're gaining weight or increasing in size again, go back to Phase I. Also, you should do interval training to increase your lean muscle mass and metabolism.

If you want to lose three or more sizes, remain on Phase I for 60 to 90 days, depending on how many sizes you would like to lose. When you're at your desired size, slowly start adding a few of the gluten-free grains into your diet and see how you do. You might find that your progress slows with the addition of the grains. If that happens, remove them from your diet again. You should also limit your servings of fruit to one serving per day until your metabolism is more stable. Focus your meals and snacks on vegetables, proteins, and healthy fats.

You might want to consider supplementation to help increase your insulin sensitivity and stabilize your adrenals. You should focus on interval training and strength training, making sure to scale the exercises appropriately to your ability. Have all your hormone levels checked—estrogen, progesterone, testosterone, DHEA, cortisol, insulin, and thyroid—to see whether there are any imbalances.

Success and Maintenance

After you reach your desired size, continue to follow all the principles of the diet. It's going to be important for you to limit stress and cortisol demand. Also, it's important for you to get adequate sleep and limit your exposure to toxins. If you find that you're continually having trouble with maintaining your desired weight or size, consider hormone testing to see whether there is an imbalance in your hormones.

The Least You Need to Know

- One shortcoming of the BMI is that is doesn't take into account the percentage of body fat versus muscle. Therefore, it's not a good indicator of true metabolism.

- After Phase I, if you find that the addition of grains back into your diet causes weight gain, remove them from your diet.

- Children and teens occasionally gain weight prior to going through a growth spurt, which should not be mistaken for overweight or obesity.

- The earlier in your life that you work at keeping your metabolism healthy, the better off you'll be.

- If you're having difficulty losing weight even though your diet is good, have your hormone levels checked to make sure that they're balanced.

Glossary

adaptogen   An herb product that is thought to increase resistance to stress, trauma, anxiety, and fatigue.

adrenal fatigue   A condition that occurs when the adrenal glands can no longer supply enough cortisol to meet the body's demands. It usually occurs after one or more episodes of chronic stress.

adrenal glands   Glands that sit on top of the kidneys. They release the hormones cortisol and adrenaline in response to stress.

aerobic capacity   The maximum capacity of an individual's body to take in and utilize oxygen during exercise, which reflects the physical fitness of the individual.

amino acids   Substances that are the building blocks for proteins and enzymes and, in times of need, glucose.

anabolic   The metabolic pathways that construct molecules from smaller units; these reactions require energy.

antibodies   Proteins that the immune system uses to fight off offenders, such as bacteria and viruses. Sometimes our body can make antibodies against its own tissues in autoimmune disease.

antioxidants   Substances that protect bodies from oxidation, or damage caused by unstable molecules called free radicals.

beta-carotene   A strongly colored red-orange pigment abundant in plants and fruits. It is the most well-known source for pro-vitamin A.

bioidentical hormones   Hormones that are identical in molecular structure to the hormones that men and women make in their bodies. Because they have the same structure, they have the ability to fit into all of the hormone receptors on the cells. They are metabolized the same way our body naturally metabolizes hormones.

Bisphenol A (BPA)   A chemical produced in large quantities for use primarily in the production of polycarbonate plastics and epoxy resins. It's a known endocrine disruptor and can create hormone imbalance either by mimicking a hormone or blocking it.

blood glucose   The amount of glucose (sugar) present in the bloodstream.

body mass index (BMI)   An approximation for human body fat based on an individual's weight and height. BMI doesn't actually measure the percentage of body fat; it's the individual's body weight divided by the square of his or her height.

C-reactive protein   A protein made in the liver in response to inflammation, it's a marker for the risk of heart inflammation and heart attack.

caffeine   A stimulant found in products such as coffee, tea, soda, and chocolate.

caffeinism   Combines caffeine dependency with a number of other symptoms such as nervousness, anxiety, insomnia, and headaches.

calorie   A unit of energy provided to the body by breaking down food into its component nutrients. Technically, it approximates the energy needed to increase the temperature of 1 gram of water by 1°C.

carotenoids   Chemicals with nutritive properties that exist in the pigment that colors plants. They are important antioxidants.

catabolic   Pathways that break down molecules into smaller units and release energy.

celiac disease   A condition that damages the lining of the small intestine and prevents it from absorbing parts of food that are important for staying healthy. The damage is due to a reaction to eating gluten, which is found in wheat, barley, and rye. It also increases the risk of autoimmune disease.

cholesterol   A waxy substance produced in bodies and found in diets. It's an essential part of cell membranes; bile acids; steroid hormones; and the fat-soluble vitamins, A, E, D, and K.

chromium   An essential nutrient involved in the regulation of carbohydrate and fat metabolism.

circuit training   Performing different exercises on different muscle groups one right after another.

colon hydrotherapy   A procedure in which warm water is gently introduced into the large intestine so waste products can be removed.

complex   Two individually charged atoms (like sodium and chloride) that bind together to form a neutral pair (sodium chloride; also known as table salt).

compound exercise   Multi-joint movements that work several muscles or muscle groups at one time. They are more beneficial than isolation exercises, where you only focus on one muscle at a time.

conscious eating   A nutrition philosophy based on the idea that listening to the body's natural hunger signals is a more effective way to reach a healthy weight than keeping track of the amount of energy and fats in foods. It's a process intended to create a healthy relationship with food, mind, and body.

CoQ10 (*co-cue-ten*)   A substance found in every cell, it's used in the reaction to produce fuel by the mitochondria, the energy-generating components of cells.

cortisol   A steroid hormone considered the "stress hormone," it comes from the adrenal gland located on top of the kidney. It helps our body respond to emergencies by increasing blood sugar, blood pressure, and heart rate. It's meant to be a short-term response.

cross-training   Doing more than one type of activity to develop fitness.

cytokines   Proteins that serve as messengers between cells and regulate inflammatory responses.

DDT (dichlorodiphenyltrichloroethane)   A well-known synthetic pesticide that was widely used from 1950 to 1980. It has been found to be related to diabetes, cancer, genetic damage, and endocrine disruption. In 1972, DDT was banned in the United States. As of 2007, India is the only country that still allows the use of DDT.

detoxification   A process by which your body transforms toxins and medications into harmless, water-soluable molecules that can be eliminated easily from your body.

down regulating receptors   A cell has receptors for things like hormones that allow it to communicate with its outside world. When there are too many hormones around the cell, it gets overwhelmed, pulls its receptors back inside, and stops communicating.

endocrine disruptors   Substances that change the way hormones are produced and the way they interact in the body.

endorphins   Chemicals produced by the body that suppress pain and make you feel good.

essential nutrients   Nutrients that the body cannot manufacture in sufficient amounts but are necessary for survival and must be taken in via food.

estrogen   A group of steroid hormones found in women and, in smaller amounts, men. There are three major types: estrone (E1), estradiol (E2), and estriol (E3). They are important for mood, sleep, memory, reproduction, heart health, and skin vitality.

fat cells   Cells that are used by the body to store excess calories (energy) for future use. Some types of fat can produce hormones and create inflammation.

fat-soluble vitamins   Vitamins stored in the fat tissue of the body and in the liver. Our fat-soluble vitamins are A, E, D, and K.

fatty acids   Acids that are usually bonded, three at a time, to a molecule called glycerol, which produces a molecule called a triglyceride.

ghrelin   A hormone that tells your brain when you are hungry.

gliadin   A glycoprotein present in wheat and several other cereals within the grass genus *Triticum*.

glucagon   A hormone made by the pancreas whose function is to raise blood sugar by releasing glucose from its storage complex, glycogen.

GLUT4 (Glucose Transporter Type 4)   A protein found in adipose tissues and striated muscle (skeletal and cardiac) that's responsible for insulin-regulated glucose translocation into the cell. In other words, GLUT4 helps glucose get into the cell.

gluten   From the Latin word for "glue," a storage protein that appears in foods processed from wheat and related species, including barley and rye. The gliadin fraction is most problematic.

gluten sensitivity   A condition in which an individual is sensitive to gluten and, when she eats it, develops irritation in her intestines that creates inflammation.

glycemic index   An indicator of how much a food will raise blood glucose (sugar) levels on its own.

glycemic load   An indicator of how much a whole meal will raise your blood glucose (sugar) level.

glycogen   Stored glucose produced by the liver.

Graves' disease (hyperthyroidism)   An autoimmune disease in which the thyroid is overactive.

green tea   Tea made with the leaves of *Camellia sinensis* that are specially treated and have undergone minimal oxidation during processing. It's a strong antioxidant.

Hashimoto's thyroiditis   An autoimmune disease in which the body makes antibodies against the thyroid and causes hypothyroidism (low thyroid function).

high-density lipoprotein (HDL)   A lipoprotein made in the liver that transports cholesterol mostly back to the liver or organs where steroid hormones are made. It's also known as "good" cholesterol because it can remove cholesterol from arterial plaques for use in hormone production.

human growth hormone (HGH)   An important hormone for overall balance in the body, HGH is produced in a small gland in the brain called the pituitary gland. The highest amounts are produced during the first 90 minutes of sleep.

hyperthyroid   An overactive thyroid.

hypothyroid   An underactive thyroid.

insulin   A hormone originating in the pancreas, its most important function is to stabilize blood sugar levels by moving sugar from the blood into muscle and fat cells.

insulin resistance   Insulin-sensitive cells have pulled back their receptors so they don't respond to insulin anymore. If you're insulin resistant, you need more insulin to keep your blood sugar levels stable.

interval training   Bursts of high-intensity exercise alternated with periods of rest.

L-carnitine   An amino acid made from lysine, methionine, niacin, vitamin B_6, iron, and vitamin C. It's very helpful for weight loss.

leptin   A hormone that tells your brain you don't need more food.

low-density lipoprotein (LDL)   A lipoprotein that enables lipids (fats) like cholesterol and triglycerides to be transported within the water-based bloodstream. It's referred to as "bad" cholesterol because higher levels of LDL are associated with increased heart disease.

melatonin   A hormone produced by the pineal gland in the brain, it's an initiator of sleep. Melatonin is a very strong antioxidant and is produced only in the dark.

menopause   The lack of menses for 12 continuous months due to ovarian failure. Estrogen levels go down for many (but not all) women at this time.

metabolism   A set of chemical reactions that happen in an organism that allow it to grow, reproduce, and respond to its environment. Metabolism can be either anabolic (building the body up) or catabolic (tearing the body down).

minerals   A chemical element that supports the biochemical reactions of metabolism with the required elemental components. They have an unequal number of electrons (negatively charged particles) and protons (positively charged particles), so they have either a positive or negative charge.

mitochondria   The powerhouses of the cell. They act like a digestive system for the cell that takes in nutrients, breaks them down, and creates energy.

neuropeptide Y   The most abundant neuropeptide in the brain. It stimulates hunger.

neuropeptides   Chemicals similar to proteins that are released by neurons (brain cells) to carry messages between cells.

nonbioidentical hormones   Hormones that are based on our body's natural hormones but have a change in the chemical structure so they can be patented. The change in structure can change the way the hormone should work in the body and the way it's metabolized. They are sometimes called synthetic hormones.

nutrients   Chemical substances in food that the body uses to support growth, tissue maintenance and repair, and ongoing health.

organic   Foods that are produced using environmentally sound methods that don't involve modern synthetic inputs.

oxidation   The interaction between oxygen molecules and other substances. This is often seen as rust and the browning of an apple that has been cut in half.

peptide YY   A hormone that's released by protein and fat intake that helps you determine when you are full.

perimenopause   A time when ovarian function starts to decline, eggs are not regularly released, and hormone imbalances like low progesterone start to occur. The hormone imbalances can cause symptoms like hot flashes, night sweats, irregular menses, and difficulty sleeping. It can last for years prior to menopause.

periodization   Planned changes in exercise to avoid burnout and enhance fitness.

persistent organic pollutants (POP)   Chemical substances that cannot be broken down in the environment.

phthalates   Esters of phthalic acid that are mainly used as plasticizers (substances added to plastics to increase their flexibility, transparency, durability, and longevity). Phthalates are known endocrine disruptors.

prebiotics   Nondigestible food ingredients that selectively stimulate the growth and/or activity of beneficial organisms in the colon.

precursor   A compound that participates in a chemical reaction to make other compounds.

pregnenolone   A hormone produced directly from cholesterol. It's the first hormone of the steroid pathway that will produce cortisol or the sex hormones DHEA, testosterone, and estrogen.

probiotics   Live, tiny living organisms such as bacteria, viruses, and yeasts which, when administered in adequate amounts, confer a health benefit on the host.

progesterone   A hormone produced from pregnenolone in the hormone pathway. It has numerous functions, including balancing estrogen, building bones, and reducing anxiety as well as being a precursor for other steroid hormones.

sarcopenia   Age-related loss of muscle mass and strength.

satiety signals   Knowing when you're full and don't need more food.

saturated fats   Fats with no double bonds. Because they lack double bonds, they're "stiffer" in structure and make cell membranes that don't function as well as membranes made with unsaturated fats like EPA and DHA.

selenium   A mineral that is an antioxidant and is required for proper thyroid function and overall wellness.

stamina   Strength of physical constitution; staying power.

steroids   A type of hormone that's derived from cholesterol and includes pregnenolone, progesterone, cortisol, DHEA, testosterone, and estrogen.

sucralose   Also known as Splenda, an artificial sweetener that has been linked to migraines and low thyroid.

testosterone   A steroid hormone produced mainly in the testes in men and in the ovaries and adrenals (in much smaller quantities) in women. It's the "life force" hormone and has many functions, including improving mood, increasing lean muscle mass, building bones, and enhancing libido.

thermogenesis   The process of heat production in warm-blooded animals. It requires energy and increases the expenditure of calories.

thyroid   One of the largest glands in the body and the only gland that stores hormones. The thyroid produces two main types of thyroid hormone, thyroxine (T4) and triidothyronine (T3), which help to increase metabolism.

thyroid hormone   A group of hormones produced by the thyroid gland to increase metabolism. The main thyroid hormone is called thyroxine (T4); another hormone, triidothyronine (T3), is produced in small amounts by the thyroid and converted from T4 in your liver and kidneys.

toxin   A poisonous substance produced by living cells or organisms.

triglycerides   Made from glycerol and three fatty acids. They're the chemical form in which most fat exists in food as well as in the body.

visceral fat   Surrounds your organs. You need some visceral fat to protect your organs. However, it is very inflammatory and is the source of the fat around our midsections (belly fat).

vitamin   An organic chemical compound that's needed for optimal function of the body. It can't be synthesized in sufficient quantities by an organism, so it must be obtained from the diet.

Resources

I made many recommendations in the book for things that you might not be used to using. Here are the best sources I've found for some of my favorite things. If you find any amazing products that help you stick to the seven principles, let me know about them at info@DrAliciaStanton.com.

Organic Food Sources

Ancient Organics (www.ancientorganics.com)   They ship organic ghee anywhere. There's also a listing of retail stores where it can be purchased.

Dagoba Organic Chocolate (www.dagobachocolate.com)   They specialize in organic dark chocolate bars, drinking chocolate, and baking chocolate. They ship throughout the United States.

Eatwild.com (www.eatwild.com)   Your source for information about safe, healthy, natural, and nutritious grass-fed beef, lamb, goats, bison, poultry, pork, dairy, and other wild edibles. Provides help with locating local farmers and farmers who ship.

Grass Fed Farms (www.grassfedfarms.com)   They supply free-range chicken and eggs as well as grass-fed beef.

Great Alaska Seafood (www.great-alaska-seafood.com)   Wild salmon, smoked salmon, giant crab legs, colossal scallops, and prawns—from the Kenai Peninsula, Alaska, to your door.

LÄRABAR (www.larabar.com)   LÄRABAR is a delicious blend of fruits, nuts, and spices—energy in its purest form. Made from 100 percent whole food, each flavor contains two to nine ingredients. Pure and simple, just as nature intended. They are gluten free, dairy free, soy free, organic, and non-GMO. The website lists retail locations and online options for purchase.

Madhava Honey (www.madhavasagave.com)   They list stores that carry their organic agave syrup and sources for online purchase and shipping as well.

Mountain Rose Herbs (www.mountainroseherbs.com)   They offer organic essential oils, herbs, and green teas. They ship their products in the United States and internationally.

Nutiva (www.nutiva.com)   They carry organic, gluten-free, dairy-free, and non-GMO coconut oil, hemp, and chia seeds. They ship all over the United States.

Seventh Generation (www.seventhgeneration.com)   They provide an extensive product line focusing on green cleaning, including disinfectants, baby products, laundry products, household cleaners, household paper and supplies, feminine care, hand wash soaps, and dishwashing soaps. They offer information for retail store locations and online purchasing.

Steaz Diet Green Tea Sodas (www.steazsoda.com)   Made with the finest organic ingredients and sweetened with the all-natural leaves of the stevia plant to create perfect refreshment for health- and weight-conscious consumers, the new line is based on Steaz's award-winning sparkling green tea formula. Steaz Zero Calorie provides 120 milligrams of natural tea antioxidants. (A personal favorite is black cherry.)

Teeccino Herbal Coffees (www.teeccino.com)   Teeccino Caffeine-Free Herbal Coffee is a delicious blend of herbs, grains, fruits, and nuts that are roasted and ground to brew and taste just like coffee.

U.S. Wellness Meats (www.grassfedbeef.com)   A collection of restaurants and retail stores (some ship) that sell grassland meats (beef, poultry, lamb, bison, etc.). They have excellent beef sticks that are nitrate free and gluten free and don't have MSG or HFCS.

Vermont Soap Organics (www.vermontsoap.com)   Vermont Soap Organics produces USDA-approved, certified-organic alternatives to the chemical- and detergent-based personal care products now in general use. They manufacture handmade bar soap for sensitive skin, the first truly organic shower gels, and organic nontoxic cleaners.

Vita Coco Coconut Water (www.vitacoco.com)   Coconut water is a natural way to hydrate and provide electrolytes. It's much better for recovery for athletes than sports drinks. This is one of my favorite brands.

White Egret Farm (www.whiteegretfarm.com)   Order information for drug-free beef, pork, and turkey as well as goat's milk and cheese.

Anti-Aging and Integrative Medicine Physicians

These are resources to help you locate a physician who focuses on nutrition and hormone balance in your area:

- American Academy of Anti-Aging (www.worldhealth.net)

- American College for the Advancement of Medicine (www.acam.org)

- BodyLogicMD (www.bodylogicmd.com)

- Fellowship for Anti-Aging and Regenerative Medicine (www.faarm.com)

- Institute of Functional Medicine (www.functionalmedicine.org)

Compounding Pharmacies

Compounding pharmacies provide a wide range of services, including custom-made prescriptions and the ability to fill prescriptions from pharmaceutical companies. It's important to use a high-quality compounding pharmacy.

Medaus (www.medaus.com)   Offers many pharmacy services, including compounding, pharmaceuticals, and nutritional supplements. Located in Birmingham, Alabama; will ship internationally.

Professional Compounding Centers of America (PCCA) (www.pccarx.com) This site offers information about some of the best compounding pharmacies in the country.

University Compounding Pharmacy (www.ucprx.com)   This site offers many pharmacy services, including compounding, pharmaceuticals, and nutritional supplements. Located in San Diego, California; will ship internationally.

Laboratory Testing Services

Laboratory tests are an important way to evaluate hormone levels, food sensitivities, level of toxin exposure, and other important aspects of your health. The following companies are the best in the business, and I use all of them for my patients' testing needs.

- ALCAT (www.alcat.com)

- Genova Diagnostics (www.genovadiagnostics.com)

- Metametrix (www.metametrix.com)

- NeuroScience (www.neurorelief.com)

- Quest Diagnostics (www.questdiagnostics.com)

- SpectraCell Laboratories (www.spectrcell.com)

- ZRT Laboratory (www.zrtlabs.com)

High-Quality Supplement Companies

I can't emphasize enough how important it is to get your supplements from a reputable source. The following companies have the highest standards for manufacturing supplements. Many of them work directly with practitioners.

- Biotics Research Corporation (www.bioticsresearch.com)

- Designs for Health (www.designsforhealth.com)

- Future Formulations, LLC (www.futureformulations.com)

- Metagenics (www.metagenics.com)

- Ortho Molecular Products (www.orthomolecularproducts.com)

- Pharmax, LLC (www.pharmaxLLC.com)

- Xymogen (www.xymogen.com)

Supplementation for Hormone-Related Health Issues

Take the test in Chapter 15 and have your hormone levels checked. If you have any issues with low thyroid, metabolic syndrome, men's hormone health, or women's hormone health, consider taking supplements, which are described in the following pages. (Information on adrenal and sleep supplementation is in Chapter 16, and information on detoxification is in Chapter 12.)

Low Thyroid (Hypothyroidism)

Low thyroid or hypothyroidism can create significant problems with metabolism and can make weight loss difficult. Hypothyroidism is a fairly common problem and becomes more common as people age. It's estimated that between one in five to one in seven people suffer from hypothyroidism. There are a vast number of things that can cause low thyroid hormone production. One of the most common is stress. Remember, cortisol, your stress hormone, reduces the conversion of your less active thyroxine (T4) to more active triiodothyronine (T3), which increases your metabolism.

Supplementation for Low Thyroid

Supplement	Daily Dose
Vitamin A	5,000 IU
B complex	100 mg
Vitamin C	1,000 mg
Vitamin D	400 IU
Zinc	25–50 mg
CoQ10	100 mg
Selenium	200 mcg
Fish oils	2,000 mg

If you require thyroid medication, it's important that you take both T4 (the less active hormone found in Synthroid and Levothroid) and T3 (the more active hormone found in Cytomel). Many physicians prescribe only Synthroid, and they rely on your body's ability to convert it to T3. Many things can hinder this conversion; you're better off taking T3 as well so you get the full benefit.

Armour Thyroid contains a combination of T4 and T3 (as well as a small amount of T2 and T1). You can also work with a compounding pharmacy to have them make you a combination of T3 and T4. You have several options to make supplementation work. Just make sure that your physician checks your levels of free T3 and free T4 and prescribes accordingly.

Metabolic Syndrome

Insulin resistance, metabolic syndrome, and diabetes are a continuum that describes an inability to handle blood sugar appropriately. With insulin resistance and metabolic syndrome, your blood sugar levels are usually still within the normal range. However, you require much more insulin to keep them in range. By the time you're diabetic, even though your body tries to use all the insulin it can, your blood sugar is elevated. The following list shows risk factors for metabolic syndrome:

- Blood pressure greater than 130/85

- Fasting blood sugar greater than 100 mg/dL

- High-density lipoprotein cholesterol (HDL) below 50 mg/dL (woman) or 40 mg/dL (man)

- Triglycerides greater than 150 mg/dL
- Waist measurement greater than 35 inches (women) or 40 inches (man)

Metabolic syndrome is diagnosed when you have three or more of the preceding risk factors. These risk factors usually indicate that you have had chronically elevated insulin levels. If you have metabolic syndrome, the risk of diabetes increases by five times, and you have twice the risk of heart disease. The good news is that following the principles of the hormone weight-loss diet will help you control your insulin response. It's also important for you to control stress and your cortisol demand.

Other important aspects of treatment for metabolic syndrome and diabetes are exercise and adequate sleep. Exercise, especially interval and weight training, increases the number of muscle cells you have. Your cells use more of your blood sugar and activate the GLUT4 transport so that your muscle cells can use sugar without even needing insulin, which reduces your insulin demand. Sleep is closely tied to insulin response.

Supplements for Metabolic Syndrome

Supplement	Daily Dose
Fish oils	2,000 mg
Zinc	25–50 mg
Alpha lipoic acid	200–600 mg
Chromium	400–600 mcg
CLA	1,000–3,000 mg
Vanadium	20–50 mg
Vitamin D	400 IU
Vitamin C	1,000 mg
Inositol	2,000–4,000 mg
B complex	100 mg

Women's Hormone Health

I've discussed many aspects of women's health throughout this book. Of course, following all the principles of the hormone weight-loss diet keeps your hormones balanced. If you're having symptoms of perimenopause, PMS, polycystic ovarian syndrome, or other female hormone-related symptoms, consider having your hormones tested and follow up with a physician to consider hormone therapy if you choose.

Remember, the key to keeping sex hormones such as estrogen, progesterone, and testosterone balanced is to manage stress and reduce your cortisol demand. The following supplement suggestions are adapted from the book *Vitamins: Hype or Hope* by Dr. Pamela Smith.

Supplementation for PMS

Supplement	Daily Dose
Fish oils	2,000 mg
Calcium	1,000 mg
Magnesium	600 mg
B complex	100 mg
Vitamin E	400 IU
Vitamin A	5,000–10,000 IU
Vitamin C	2,000 mg
L-carnitine	500 mg
Chromium	400 mcg
Inositol	500 mg

Supplementation for Polycystic Ovarian Syndrome

Supplement	Daily Dose
Fish oils	2,000 mg
Inositol	1,000 mg
Chromium	1,000 mg
Vanadium	50 mg
Zinc	25–50 mg
L-carnitine	1,000–6,000 mg
Alpha lipoic acid	500 mg
B complex	100 mg
Magnesium	600 mg
Vitamin D	1,000 IU
Vitamin C	2,000 mg

Supplements for Those Using Birth Control Pills or Hormone Replacement Therapy

Supplement	Daily Dose
Inositol	1,000 mg
Magnesium	600 mg
Alpha lipoic acid	500 mg
L-carnitine	1,000 mg
Phosphatidyl choline	2,000 mg
B complex	100 mg

Men's Hormone Health

A man's testosterone production peaks in his 20s. After that time, testosterone production starts decreasing approximately 1 percent per year. In addition, stress and insulin resistance can add belly fat, which causes the conversion of testosterone to estrogen and the production of a protein in the liver called sex hormone binding globulin (SHBG). SHBG is designed to pick up extra estrogen. However, it also binds with testosterone. The combination of lower testosterone production, increased testosterone conversion to estrogen, and increased binding of testosterone by SHBG can create symptoms of low testosterone in men. The following is a list of symptoms of low testosterone in men:

- Decreased muscle mass
- Depression
- Difficulty sleeping
- Erectile dysfunction
- Fatigue
- High cholesterol
- Low libido

The principles of the hormone weight-loss diet help you maintain your testosterone level. However, if the symptoms are significant, you should have your hormone levels checked and follow up with a physician to consider testosterone therapy. Exercise, especially interval training and strength training, naturally increase testosterone levels. It's also important to limit your exposure to toxins, such as Bisphenol A (BPA) and phthalates, because they are antitestosterone.

Supplementation for Low Testosterone in Men

Supplement	Daily Dose
Zinc	35–50 mg
Copper	1–2 mg
Saw palmetto	320 mg
Selenium	200 mcg
Vitamin B complex	100 mg
Flaxseed	1,000 mg
GLA	500 mg
Vitamin A	5,000 IU
Vitamin C	1,000 mg

Personal Action Plan Worksheets

This appendix provides and explains how to use three personal action worksheets that will help you create an action plan for your weight loss. The worksheets can also be downloaded at www.DrAliciaStanton.com.

Worksheet #1: Monthly Measurement Monitor

This sheet is meant to be used once a month so you can really follow your progress. The goal is to get your measurements written down before you start Phase I and to see what some of your baseline exercises would be. If you can, it's also a great idea to have photographs taken from the front and the side so you can see your progress.

Chest measurement: Wrap the tape measure around your chest, holding the ends in front. It should lie just under your arms, across your shoulder blades, and across the fullest part of your chest (above your breasts for women).

Arm measurement: For the biceps measurement, measure your arm at the fullest part. For consistency each month, you might want to measure a certain distance from your elbow or down from your shoulder.

Waist measurement: Your waist measurement reflects the narrowest part of your waist. For most women, this is about an inch above the belly button.

Hip measurement: Your hip measurement usually reflects the fullest part of your hips, so it's roughly the area you sit on.

Thigh measurement: Measure your thighs where they are the largest. For consistency each month, you might want to measure down from your groin the same number of inches and then measure the circumference of your thigh from that point.

Exercise: For the exercise portion of the worksheet, write down any times that you have from the timed workouts. For workouts, write down the number of rounds you completed. You might also want to write down whether you did basic movements, intermediate movements, or advanced movements so you can track your progress.

Personal Action Plan Worksheet #1
Monthly Measurement Monitor

Beginning Date: _____ End Date: _____

Diet: Phase I _____ Phase II _____

	Beginning of Month	End of Month
Body fat percentage:	_____	_____
Weight:	_____	_____
Measurement:		
Chest	_____	_____
Right arm	_____	_____
Left arm	_____	_____
Waist	_____	_____
Hips	_____	_____
Left thigh	_____	_____
Right thigh	_____	_____
Tabata squat score	_____	_____
Tabata pushup score	_____	_____
Tabata sit-up score	_____	_____
Rounds workout #1	_____	_____
Time for workout #2	_____	_____
Time for workout #3	_____	_____
Rounds workout #4	_____	_____
Time for workout #5	_____	_____
Time for workout #6	_____	_____

Worksheet #2: Daily Monitor—Stress Management and Exercise

This is one of the two worksheets you will use every day. The top part focuses on stress management and sleep. You begin with your gratitude journal by writing down three things for which you're grateful. This worksheet also helps you to monitor your energy level throughout the day. I usually tell my patients to mark down their energy levels on a scale of 1 to 10. A score of 10 is the most energy—in other words, you're on top of the world. A score of 1 is dead tired; you can barely get out of bed. Write down how many hours of sleep you got last night and what time you're planning to be in bed tonight.

These worksheets will help to determine possible problems with your diet or lifestyle. If you're consistently writing down that you're getting only five hours of sleep a night, that's a problem. You should be as honest as you can on these worksheets because the information you write down can be very helpful in determining why things are or aren't working for you.

It's important to plan something specific to do for stress relief each day. Make sure you find time at least three times every day to stop and take five deep breaths. Write down what you're doing when you stop to do it. If it's during a stressful situation, write down whether it makes a difference or not.

For the exercise portion, write down the elements of the workout(s) you plan to do. Also, if you're to do a certain number of rounds (i.e., five rounds of three different exercises), write down the time it takes you to complete the specified number of rounds. If you're supposed to do as many rounds as possible during a given time (5 minutes, 10 minutes, etc.), write down the number of rounds you complete in the allotted time.

Personal Action Plan Worksheet #2

Daily Monitor—Stress Management and Exercise

Today's Date: _____   Phase: _____   Day #: _____

Gratitude: Three things I'm thankful for today

1.

2.

3.

Energy level when I woke up this morning: _____ noon _____ evening _____ night _____

How many hours of sleep did I get last night? _____

My planned bedtime tonight is: _____

Stress Relief: What did I do for myself today?

Stop and take five deep breaths at least three times today. What were you doing at the time you did them?

1.

2.

3.

Exercise Today:

Workout:

_____

_____

_____

Time: _____ Number of rounds completed: _____

Today, my workout felt:

_____

I was held accountable by:

_____

Worksheet #3: Daily Monitor—Diet

It's been proven that if you keep a food diary and document what you're eating, you're much more likely to lose weight. This worksheet starts by asking whether there are any challenges such as traveling, illness, or other unexpected issues. Next, write down what you eat for your meals and snacks. If you tried a new recipe that you liked or found one that you want to try, write that down so you remember it. There's also an area to document your supplement and water intake. Write down the number of times each day you actually get thirsty, which will eventually help you remember to drink water more consistently.

This worksheet also allows you to plan your meals for the next day and jot down anything you may need to pick up at the grocery store. Last but not least, think about how you're eating. Are you conscious? Are your emotions beneficial for your overall goals? To whom were you accountable?

Personal Action Plan Worksheet #3

Daily Monitor—Diet

Date: _____   Phase: _____   Day #: _____

Meal challenges I had today:

_____

_____

Breakfast:

_____

_____

Mid-morning snack:

_____

Lunch:

_____

_____

Mid-afternoon snack:

_____

Dinner:

_____

_____

Water intake: _____ How many times was I thirsty today? _____

Supplements: Multivitamin: _____ Fish oil: _____
Vitamin D: _____

Others:

_____

Meal plans for tomorrow:

_____

Shopping list:

_____

_____

_____

New recipe that I loved today:

_____

Did I eat consciously today?

_____

Did I monitor my portion sizes and servings?

_____

Were my emotions beneficial to me today?

_____

Today, I felt:

_____

Q and A with Dr. Stanton

I get questions from my patients every day regarding all aspects of their health. I wanted to share with you the most common questions I get regarding diet and my answers to those questions. If you have other questions, send them to me at info@ DrAliciaStanton.com.

Question: I am 40 years old and need to lose 45 pounds. I have tried many very low-calorie diets and am afraid that I have damaged my metabolism. The weight is now coming off very slowly. What do you think?

Answer: Although the very-low-calorie starvation diet cycle can damage your metabolism and reduce your basal metabolic rate, it's definitely possible to restore them. However, it took a while for you to damage your metabolism, and it will take a while to repair it.

When you start eating whole foods and stop eating metabolism-damaging processed foods and trans fats, you'll start to heal. By implementing interval and strength training, you'll increase your lean muscle mass, which also increases your metabolism. I recommend that you have your hormone levels tested so you can see whether there's a problem with your thyroid gland. Over time, with your increased lean muscle mass and increased metabolism, you'll lose weight, and more importantly, you'll reduce your size and have a healthy, lean body.

Question: Can I drink fruit juices?

Answer: I don't recommend drinking fruit juices because they're very high in sugar and don't contain any fiber. Therefore, the sugar rapidly enters your bloodstream, causing a high insulin demand. Technically, tomato juice is a fruit juice, but I recommend it because it has far less sugar than fruit juices. Also, you can drink beet and carrot juices if you choose, but they have a little bit more sugar.

Question: Should I eat egg whites instead of whole eggs?

Answer: You can eat the entire egg, yolk and white. It has been shown that eating the cholesterol in the egg yolk will not raise your cholesterol levels. In addition, the yolks have omega-3 fatty acids that are helpful in fighting inflammation. Make sure you eat organic eggs, which have not been exposed to hormones or antibiotics.

Question: What about an egg substitute?

Answer: There's nothing wrong with real eggs, especially organic eggs. There's no reason to substitute healthy, omega-3 fatty acid filled eggs with a substitute.

Question: I've heard that as I get older (I'm 55), I'll need to eat less calories or I'll gain weight. How do I maintain your diet plan on fewer calories? I'll be hungry all the time!

Answer: The main reason you need fewer calories as you get older is that you naturally decrease the amount of lean muscle mass you have as you age. Therefore, with less muscle mass, your metabolism slows down, so you need fewer calories. One right way to combat the natural decrease in muscle mass is to do interval and strength training.

I don't focus on calories with this diet plan. You'll be allowed to eat healthy, whole foods containing unrefined carbohydrates, proteins, and healthy fats. These foods also contain a lot of natural fiber. The proteins, fats, and fiber will help fill you up. On top of that, they'll help you control your appetite hormones, leptin and ghrelin, which will do even more to help you feel full. Remember to make sure that you're drinking enough water as well, since thirst can be mistaken for hunger. Also, because you'll be eating in a manner that will help balance insulin, you'll also help balance cortisol. This will reduce your level of belly fat and any extra breakdown of protein or muscle normally caused by high cortisol.

Question: Is low-fat milk okay? What about fat-free half-and-half?

Answer: Because milk contains a number of potential allergens, dairy products are not allowed in Phase I of the program. This will allow your body to reduce the amount of inflammation it has and help your metabolism heal. In Phase II, you can add dairy products back into your diet and see how you feel. You may find that you have a sensitivity to dairy products and notice things like bloating, gas, weight gain, sinus congestion, or a number of other symptoms. In that case, remove the dairy products from your diet again and add almond milk or coconut milk to your diet. If you find that you can tolerate dairy products, I would prefer that you use full-fat products.

The natural fat that you find in milk is actually healthy. As a matter of fact, the fat in milk plays a role in weight loss. Milk fat contains conjugated linoleic acid (CLA), which promotes weight loss, vitamins, and a compound that can raise high-density lipoprotein cholesterol (HDL, the good kind). When the fat is removed from the milk, these healthy ingredients are removed and replaced with sugar. Therefore, you actually increase your blood sugar and insulin demand when you use low-fat or fat-free dairy products.

Question: Do you recommend foods made by Weight Watchers, Nutrisystem, Atkins, or Jenny Craig?

Answer: Many of the foods produced by these companies contain added chemicals, artificial sweeteners, and partially hydrogenated oils. These additives can wreak havoc on your hormones, which will only set you back on your goal of healing your metabolism and losing weight. In addition, some of these diets monitor food only by calorie counts, and not by the nutritional value of the ingredients. The lack of nutrients can lead to significant problems in the long run. I focus on whole, healthy foods in my diet because you'll not only lose weight, you'll be healthier.

Question: I am past menopause, and I don't want to take hormones. However, I have a lot of belly fat even though I exercise. What can I do?

Answer: Many times, the increased belly fat is due to excess cortisol. You may have excess cortisol because of stress, eating a diet that doesn't provide a steady blood sugar, having food sensitivities, or having a chronic infection. The excess cortisol can also cause an imbalance with your other hormones. Therefore, if you don't want to take hormones, the best way to keep them in balance is to follow the seven principles of my diet, focusing especially on stress reduction to lower cortisol demand.

Question: What is the glycemic index of nongluten breads and pastas?

Answer: Pastas made with white rice don't contain gluten but may have a high glycemic index. I recommend that you utilize whole grains that are gluten free, such as brown rice and quinoa. Remember, you can reduce the insulin impact of a food by reducing its glycemic load. Eating a little fat with nongluten foods, such as olive oil or almond butter, will do the trick. (Even though the glycemic index of one part of the meal may be a little bit higher, the impact of the whole meal on your blood sugar will not be as significant.)

Question: After I am on the maintenance diet, how often should I have my hormones checked?

Answer: I recommend getting a baseline set of labs done to look at all of your hormones and other important values, such as homocysteine and highly sensitive C-reactive protein, when you start the maintenance program. If your labs look good and you don't have any major symptoms, you may not need to get your hormones tested very often. However, if you're having symptoms or your initial laboratory values were not optimal, I would check your hormone levels every six months or so until you feel better or your lab values are in the optimal range.

Question: What would you recommend for insomnia? Do you think prescription aids are alright long term?

Answer: Occasionally, if I have a patient in an extremely stressful situation, or one who has significant difficulty sleeping despite using supplements, I'll suggest a prescription sleep aid for a short time. At the same time, I work with the patient to reduce his stress levels, improve his diet and lifestyle, and increase his exercise so he can move toward improving his sleep on his own. I like to limit the use of prescription sleep aids as much as possible and would rather not have patients on them long term.

Question: Will my skin break out on this diet?

Answer: Initially, as your body begins to detox and removes toxins, you may have some mild breakouts. This is because your skin is the mirror of what is happening within your body. As your body adjusts to a healthy diet, your skin should improve significantly. Many processed foods, trans fats, and chemical additives have a negative impact on your skin. Therefore, if you remove these things and eat whole foods that are rich in vitamins and nutrients, your skin will benefit.

Question: Will I be constipated on this diet? If so, what can I do?

Answer: This diet is loaded with fiber. Many fresh vegetables and fruits contain enough fiber to keep you from being constipated. In addition, by following the seven principles of the diet, you reduce your stress levels, which will naturally enhance your thyroid function. A poorly functioning thyroid is a very common cause of constipation. By improving thyroid function, you'll reduce constipation. Also, make sure that you're drinking enough water because that will also reduce the incidence of constipation.

Question: I'm addicted to chocolate. How often can I have it as one of my special treats?

Answer: The good news is that chocolate can actually be healthy for you! Scientists at Cornell University showed that the cocoa found in chocolate has lots of antioxidants. As a matter of fact, cocoa has twice as many antioxidants as red wine and three times the amount found in green tea. Organic dark chocolate made of at least 70 percent cocoa is the best choice for your chocolate addiction. However, be very careful about the amount of sugar in some commercial chocolates. Also, make sure they're not highly processed and don't contain partially hydrogenated oil. Real organic dark chocolate made with cocoa butter will satisfy you and give you extra antioxidants. If you find chocolate that has little or no added sugar, you can have a little bit every day (1 ounce) if that'll help you stay on the rest of the diet.

Question: Can I have diet soda?

Answer: There's no place in this diet for diet soda, as the artificial sweeteners don't support hormone health and weight loss. In addition, the phosphates found in sodas leach calcium from your bones, and the Bisphenol A (BPA) that lines the cans also creates problems with your hormones.

Question: Is this diet safe for overweight children?

Answer: This is an excellent diet for overweight children. As a matter of fact, all seven principles will help them, especially stress management and appropriate sleep. Those habits, when learned early, will make a difference later in life. A diet of whole foods—including lean proteins, unrefined carbohydrates, fruits, vegetables, and healthy fats—is fantastic for any child, especially an overweight one.

Question: I need to work night shifts. Can I still follow the diet?

Answer: This diet will be especially appropriate for you because you need to make sure your blood sugars are stable. By working night shifts, you increase your risk of insulin resistance. The Centers for Disease Control recently correlated working night shifts with an increase in cancer risk. But if you focus on optimal diet, stress reduction, exercise, and adequate sleep, you may be able to reduce your risk. The easiest way to make this work is to switch your meals to match your schedule. When you're done with work, go to bed when you get home, have your "breakfast" meal when you wake up in the afternoon or evening, and follow with lunch and dinner according to your adjusted schedule.

Index